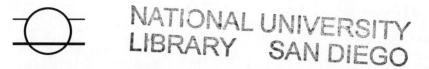
STRUGGLES FOR INCLUSIVE EDUCATION
An ethnographic study

Anastasia D. Vlachou

Open University Press
Buckingham · Philadelphia

Open University Press
Celtic Court
22 Ballmoor
Buckingham
MK18 1XW

and
1900 Frost Road, Suite 101
Bristol, PA 19007, USA

First Published 1997

A catalogue record of this book is available from the British Library

ISBN 0 335 19763 9 (pb)   0 335 19764 7 (hb)

Library of Congress Cataloging-in-Publication Data
Vlachou, Anastasia D., 1966–
    Struggles for inclusive education: an ethnographic study /
Anastasia D. Vlachou.
        p.   cm.
    Includes bibliographical references and index.
    ISBN 0-335-19764-7 (hb). – ISBN 0-335-19763-9 (pb)
    1. Inclusive education–Great Britain–Case studies.   2. Mainstreaming in education–Great Britain–Case studies.   3. Ethnic attitudes–Great Britain–Case studies.   4. Learning disabled children–Education (Elementary)–Great Britain–Case studies.   I. Title.
LC1203.G7V53   1997
371.9\046\00941–dc21   96-45150
                                                                                        CIP

Typeset by Type Study, Scarborough
Printed in Great Britain by Biddles Ltd, Guildford and King's Lynn

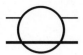

Contents

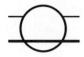

Series editor's preface

The Disability, Human Rights and Society Series reflects a commitment to a social model of disability and a desire to make this view accessible to a wide audience. 'Disability' is viewed as a form of oppression and the fundamental issue is not one of an individual's inabilities or limitations, but rather a hostile and unadaptive society.

Priority is given to identifying and challenging those barriers to change, including the urgent task of establishing links with other marginalized groups and thus seeking to make connections between class, gender, race, age and disability factors.

The series aims to further establish disability as a serious topic of study, one in which the latest research findings and ideas can be seriously engaged with.

In this informative and stimulating account of an ethnographic study, Vlachou provides the reader with a series of rich and detailed insights into the position and experiences of a primary school during a period of immense change. It is a valuable historical record of a particular school at a specific period in time, endeavouring to engage with a range of demands within a general context in which the governance, financing and functions of schools were being fundamentally re-structured.

Vlachou powerfully reminds the reader of the centrality of understanding the context and work culture in which teachers and pupils interact. This is essential if the complex and contentious nature of the conceptual and inter-actional factors are to be adequately engaged with. Part of this involves resisting the pressure to make quick and superficial interpretations of manifestly complicated intentions, actions and interactions of the participants and the wider socio-economic and ideological factors involved.

Arising from extensive observations and interviews with teachers and pupils, the author presents a challenging account of the voices and experiences of the research participants. A critique of key terms including 'disability', 'attitudes', 'normalization', 'special needs' and 'integration', provides the framework within which practices are sensitively examined.

A particularly powerful feature of the book is the material dealing with pupil perspectives. Vlachou has provided some original insights through sensitively engaging with the subtleties of interpersonal relationships between disabled and non-disabled children, of how pupils create friendships and develop meanings in relation to definitions of disability and integration.

This is an important book which offers a detailed and innovatory analysis of several key issues including disabling barriers. It both adds to our understanding and provides a strong stimulus for further debate and exploration.

Professor Len Barton
Sheffield

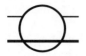

Preface

In society, responses to disability are very often accompanied by feelings of guilt, embarrassment and assumptions that disability is necessarily of negative value. Consequently disabled children experience isolation and marginalization; often we hastily assume that this is a 'natural' consequence of their specific impairments. On the other hand it has been reported that the inclusion of disabled children in ordinary schooling communities presupposes a change of attitudes. How can we explain such differences in responses? Conventional attitudinal research has been based on the assumption that the attitudes expressed by people involved directly and/or indirectly with disabled children will influence their behaviour towards the children. The importance of attitudes in the creation of more inclusive communities has thus been acknowledged, yet exploration of the nature of those attitudes has been divorced either from the wider set of social formations or from the educational context within which they have developed. My engagement with disability issues has convinced me that there is an urgent need for disability to be understood as part of a wider set of inequalities and institutionalized social formations/relations which perpetuate exclusive ideologies and practices.

Thus this book is an attempt to offer a detailed analysis of primary school teachers' and peers' attitudes towards integration; particularly, it locates the question of inclusive education within the wider educational context. A sociopolitical approach to attitudes is used because it provides the possibility of adequately addressing the complex and contradictory issues involved.

The findings presented in this book show that integration has become a contentious notion. The discussions of teachers' and peers' value conflicts and ethical dilemmas, as well as the structural conditions within which integration is implemented, attempt to show the nature and intensity of the struggles to pursue inclusive priorities. Further, the exploration of the meanings teachers and peers ascribe to their interactional and perceptual patternings with disabled pupils reveals the ways 'handicapped' identities are socially created.

This book is part of a wider struggle – which has been initiated by disabled people and their advocates – for the identification of disabling barriers and the creation of more enabling environments. It is hoped that the insights offered in this book will contribute in the quest to understand the nature of the educational enterprise within which weaker social groups continue to experience discrimination and exclusion. These insights will hopefully enable us to resist romantic notions of change and to provide teachers with the support to which they are entitled and which is necessary if laudable rhetoric is to become reality.

Anastasia D. Vlachou
Athens, Greece

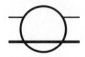

Acknowledgements

The creation of this book has been the result of five very intensive and challenging years of research work, reading and reflective thinking. Thus it is important to mention that without help and encouragement from a number of individuals the completion of this book would not have been possible.

First of all, I would like to express my gratitude to the teachers and the pupils of the school in which I undertook the research presented here, for their friendly and cooperative spirit with which they responded to my intrusion into their lives. Their contribution provided me with the invaluable opportunity to learn a lot from their experience and thoughts, and to pursue this study. Naturally, I have adopted pseudonyms for them to protect their anonymity.

I also want to express my gratitude to Professor Len Barton, for his continuous, tangible support and encouragement throughout this work. Our discussions proved to be the most valuable experience in the evolution of my thinking.

To my good friends Dimitra, Vicki, Rachel, John, Esmeralda and Yvon, with whom I have shared a variety of experiences and feelings throughout this work, I owe a heartfelt thanks.

I am also grateful to the English Language School for their substantial contribution in helping me transfer my Greek thoughts into proper English. Particularly, I am thankful for the expert assistance of Kevin, Cilla and Frances. I would like to thank the State Scholarships Foundation in Athens, because without their financial support I would not have been able to pursue one of my dreams.

Last, but very importantly, I owe a great deal to my family. To Constantinos for his 'critical eye', his selfless emotional support and encouragement, I owe a big 'ευχαριστώ'.

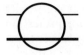

Introduction

During my early socialization process, disabled children were not children to be friends with. Whenever, accidentally, they happened to be around they were targets of jokes, objects of curiosity and pity, and provokers of fear for the 'unfortunate tricks that life can play'. Disability had better remain hidden because it was associated with feelings of guilt and embarrassment. Inclusive education was not the type of pedagogy I encountered in my schooling experience as a student, and friendships with disabled people were far from being an ordinary and typical life occurrence. The ideology of the educational system that I had experienced was based on highly competitive routes, centralized national directives, and subject-centred practices in which the student in order to succeed had to strive for 'excellence' (as it was predefined by the educational apparatus). Excellence was perceived as an individualized triumph and so was failure. In such a system disabled students simply had no place. It was not a surprise, then, that I had a cultural, ideological and educational shock some years later, working in a different educational-ethnic (Canadian) system: I experienced, as a volunteer educational psychologist, an 'integrated setting' that catered for children with a wide variety of strengths and weaknesses, including children with Down's Syndrome. The emerging question, surrounded by both doubts and puzzlement, seemed to be unavoidable: why was it that what was perceived as unfeasible – an absurd idea – in one context was feasible in another?

The above brief autobiographical account is highly relevant to this study, in which the main interest is to explore primary school teachers' and peers' attitudes towards the process of integration, with particular reference to the integration of pupils with Down's Syndrome. It constitutes an essential part of the cultural, historical and political baggage (including tensions, conflicts and enlightenment) that I, as a researcher, carried and experienced throughout the writing of this book. Often, as far as the social relations of research production are concerned, it has been ignored that 'We [the researchers] do not come innocent to a research or a situation of events; rather we situate these events not merely in the institutional meaning which our profession provides but also constitute them as expressions of ourselves' (Clough 1995: 138). Of course this element entails a risk as well, as for when the study is in the public arena,

> the researcher loses control over how it is viewed and responded to by individuals or organisations. This raises the possibility that insights are used for purposes the researcher never intended and strongly disagrees with. This is a particularly serious issue in relation to those subjects of study who are oppressed and experience institutional discrimination.
>
> (Clough 1995: 145; see also Hammersley and Scarth 1993)

In addition to risks, attitudinal research in the area of special educational needs raises serious questions about the area of special educational research policy and practice. This type of research can be one of the most difficult and demanding aspects of education and other social research. As Bines (1995: 42) pin-points, 'the researcher must confront a range of issues and dilemmas, together with many personal and social values and vested interests'. Conversely, exploring attitudes is a highly problematic affair due to the nature of the construct and the way it has been perceived and analysed in previous mainly conventional research. Basic questions have to be answered, like: What do attitudes involve? Is their formation so abstract and far apart from specific societal well-internalized norms and directives? What is the socio-political function of the 'other' in attitudinal research? Are the expressed attitudes influenced by the nature of our questioning? How are we to perceive and interpret the inconsistencies and conflicts that are to be found between expressed attitudinal statements and actions? What is the point of reference when asking about the other's attitudes: the disabled person, or the environment in which this person is called to live? Can such dichotomies exist within contexts that are based on webs of social relationships? Can we talk about situational attitudes or can we ascribe to attitudes an inherent stability regardless of situational parameters? Is there any use in studying attitudes in the first place, and if so, what are the implications for the lives of those most affected by such a type of research? These are crucial, conflicting and often confusing issues; obviously tackling such issues entails an engagement with and sensitivity to the complexity that is to be found within the realities of both the researcher and the participants.

Additionally, in the area of special educational needs the way we conceptualize the term 'attitudes' encompasses an extension to the way we conceptualize the term 'disability'. A major issue of analysis in attitudinal research is the way the notion of impairment becomes synonymous with disability. The researcher, if not engaged in continuous critical reflection upon his/her own attitudes, shares the responsibility of perpetuating this phenomenon whereby socially created assumptions are considered to be natural life occurrences.

The image of a researcher who is detached and above the environment that s/he is attempting to understand contradicts my experience, in which most

decisions emerged in the field and were based on trials, errors and recon-
structions. It has been the experience of errors and the search for alternative
ways that have helped me to realize how subjective and value-laden both the
researcher and the techniques can be, and also to realize the value of the
following statement:

> to keep our options secret, to conceal them in the cobwebs of technique,
> or to disguise them by claiming neutrality does not constitute neutrality
> ... It's naive to consider our roles as abstract in a matrix of neutral
> methods and techniques for action that doesn't take place in a neutral
> society.
>
> (Freire 1985: 39)

Further, since I am a non-British citizen and do not have first-hand experience of being educated in the British educational system, I had to approach
each situation inside and outside the classroom from a 'cultural anthropology'
stance – I had to question what for other people, who have grown up in this
specific culture, seemed to be unquestionable. This stance enabled me to
acknowledge the cultural relativity of my (Greek) society and British society,
while at the same time urging me 'to look with renewed attention at the
details which make up the "natural" attitudes of everyday life' (Webster 1980:
47).

Thus the complexities of the notions I engaged with and the unavoidable
anthropological stance that has to be adopted in a personal endeavour to give
meaning to experience(s) demanded the 'application' of methods which allow
the self to be situated into a context (see also: Freilich 1977; Cohen and
Mannion 1980; Burgess 1981, 1982, 1984, 1985; Amabile and Stubbs 1982;
Becker and Geer 1982; Gans 1982; Atkinson 1992). Ethnographic methodol-
ogy provides the space and flexibility to embrace the notion of cultural contexts and to grasp – or at least try to understand – 'other cultures on their
own terms and to identify cultural patterns within the processes of both continuity and change' (Peters 1995: 63; see also Becker and Geer 1982; Easterday *et al.* 1982; Frankenberg 1982; Delamont and Hamilton 1986; Delamont
1992) without denying that the researcher is included in the method of analysis. As Ball (1994: 4) maintains, 'ethnography is a way of engaging critically
with and developing interpretations of the "real". Like genealogy it is disruptive, it is often about giving voice to the unheard, it is also about the play of
power-knowledge relations in local and specific settings.'

The notion of 'setting' and/or the 'context' is important. The adoption of
an ethnographic approach to the study of attitudes towards the process of
integration is connected with a need to explore the context in which questions relating to disability are raised. In turn this demand is based on the realization that attitudes are 'grounded in the choices (people make) when faced
with the practical [and ideological] challenges [and constraints] of everyday
living' (Peters 1995: 65). This perspective provides a means of grasping contradictions within and between policies and practices, and understanding
'those unintended consequences that combine to provide the possibilities for

contestation and change' (Barton 1991: 3). Thus instead of conceptualizing attitudes as ahistorical, apolitical and asocial entities, in this study they are used as the means of exploring the practices and ideologies that hinder or promote the creation of more-inclusive education. They are also used as a starting point in understanding the reality of everyday life within an educational setting, in which a collection of people try to make sense of this reality, their relationships, and the tensions between themselves and their everyday educational life. We need to consider the micropolitical struggles involved in people's individual or collective efforts to pursue their goals, the ways they operate from within unequal power relationships, and the process whereby they affect and are affected by political decisions made at different levels. In relation to questions of disability, the contextual perspective of exploring attitudes offers the means to highlight the nature and intensity of the struggles over definitions, effective policy and practice (Barton 1988, 1989, 1991, 1995). For me, this perspective has found added strength and significance through the personal effort and ideological evolution involved in the processes and practices of this study, which has led to a realization that 'the idea of special educational needs is one instance of a range of categories which oppress disabled people' (Fulcher 1995: 9). This assumption can be understood only in relation to schools' wider socio-economic context.

Educational ideologies, social and cultural values are very important in any analysis of the discourses surrounding the area of special educational needs, for they underlie the structures and constraints shaping both teachers' and peers' attitudes towards the process of integration. Such an analysis is particularly urgent during an era of radical transformation, when industrial and economic preoccupations occupy the centre ground of educational politics. Of course, educational activity is one of the many social entities that cannot be examined in isolation. Schooling interconnects with a more extensive and complex reality, reflecting continual changes and transformations with unpredictable outcomes. Indeed, the character of school activity is not only a mirror of aspects of contemporary modes of production, dominant economic priorities and political activities. Education is also, as Apple (1979: 42) maintains, 'both a "cause" and an "effect". The school is not a passive mirror, but an active force, one that also serves to give legitimacy to economic and social forms and ideologies so intimately connected to it.'

This dialectical connection between school and other social systems and structures has been the starting point of raising different and even conflicting ideologies of education, its function, uses and aims. However, for over a decade there has been remorseless pressure by government to impose changes on schools and teachers through the introduction of a plethora of policies and innovations covering all aspects of educational provision and practice. Currently, state-funded schools in the UK are faced with a reform package which, in addition to introducing a national curriculum, makes wholesale changes in a number of important areas: the organization of classrooms and the teaching/learning processes, accompanied by specific ideological philosophies (see Alexander *et al.* 1993); the roles and power(s) of local educational authorities; the management, funding and governance of schools; the nature, aim and purpose of student assessments; the relationships among schools and between schools and parents; school inspection; and teachers' education, training, work conditions and professional identities (see Alexander *et al.* 1993; Hargreaves 1993; Ball 1994; Ball *et al.* 1994; Black 1994; Bolton 1994; O'Hear 1994; Pollard *et al.* 1994). In other words, schools are having to adjust to sweeping changes in the purpose, aim, function and nature of both schooling and pedagogy.

The central feature of this transformation period is the political commitment to market forces and competition as a means of increasing educational productivity. Commercial rather than educational principles are dominating political discourses, surrounded by significant shifts in the value base of educational practice. It has become difficult to differentiate the rhetoric from the realities, and while the dominant discourses give emphasis to 'choice', they often ignore the significant differences that exist between 'choosing (making a choice) and getting your choice' (Ball 1994: 23). Meanwhile, the vision encapsulated within the current political ideology of education implies that 'The best quality education is a positional good which must be rationed and competitively sought after. Values of competitive individualism, separation and exclusion are extolled and knowledge is itself regarded as a commodity for private consumption' (Tomlinson 1994: 4).

The values that define and underpin the new educational reforms and the way these reforms were introduced – if not imposed – raise fundamental concerns regarding inclusive education. Questions of equality and social justice seem to be 'outdated' in a context where the prevailing ethos values individualism, commercialism, productivity, competition and control/regulation. Many have voiced fears that within this climate it is unlikely that schools will give priority to inclusive values and comprehensive principles (Carr and Quicke 1990; Barton and Oliver 1992; Ball 1994).

Against this background (as extensively discussed in following chapters) this study endeavours to understand the question of inclusive education by exploring the context within which teachers' and peers' attitudes towards the process of integration have been developed. The research took place at a Northern primary school. The school was in an area consisting of mainly white British working class, lower middle class and middle class people. According to teachers the children came from a wide socio-economic background. Because of the development of the catchment area and the building of new council housing, a lot of new families had arrived over the last 10 to 15 years. Specifically, during 1993/4 there were 25 new children registered at the school. Teachers perceived this as problematic because the children had additional difficulties in adjusting to a new educational environment and establishing relationships with their new peers and teachers. Moreover, teachers, especially in the infants school, believed they had to deal with more complex social problems than previous years, problems originating from the high numbers of children coming from broken or extended families with low financial support.

Some of the aims of the school, as reported in official documents given to parents, were:

- to create an environment and atmosphere which will foster in the children a positive attitude to education and to life in general;
- to help pupils to develop intellectually and socially, placing a high value on literacy, numeracy and communication skills;
- to stimulate lively and enquiring minds; and
- to create an atmosphere of trust and respect in which children and adults can live and work together in a positive and supportive manner.

In pursuit of these aims it was claimed that the school was 'run on a firm, fair and friendly basis'.

The two-level building was in the middle of a huge green yard. The whole ground floor was the infants school, which catered for approximately 160 children aged 4 to 6+; it had its own playground separated from the middle school's playground. The middle school was on the top floor and catered for approximately 190 pupils aged 7 to 11+ (Year 3 up to Year 7). It was claimed by teachers, in both the infants and middle school, that the number of enrolments was increasing. In each class there were approximately 30 students, and each class included a combination of two-year age groups (i.e. Year 3 and Year 4 pupils were being educated together in one class).

The administrative aspect of the school was important. Each school, (infants and middle) had different head teachers: a female for the infants and a male head teacher for the middle school. The staffing of the infants school was made up of 13 teachers, all female except for only one male, who functioned as the head of the special needs area. Nine of the 13 were mainstream teachers; while the others functioned as resource teachers or child care assistants inside a mainstream class, or had complete responsibility for pupils with learning difficulties/disabilities in the resource room for considerable periods of time. The staffing of the middle school was made up of 11 (five female and six male) teachers. Six of the 11 were mainstream teachers, one of whom (male) additionally functioned as deputy head. The remaining five (two male and three female) were the resource teachers, being responsible mainly for the pupils with learning difficulties/disabilities.

The middle school became a junior school in 1992/3, when Year 7 was abolished. Simultaneously, both the infants and the junior school were put under one administration, with one male head teacher and two – a male and a female – deputy heads.

Within this setting I endeavoured to understand the way this collection of people interpreted their reality. Of course, what is being presented in this book is only a snapshot of a historical period in the life of this primary school. It is important to note that the data discussed in this book were collected during the years of 1992 and 1993, which can be considered as the initial phase of implementing the National Curriculum requirements. Every change involves pain, conflict and confusion, and even though policies can be 'crude and simple, practice is sophisticated, contingent, complex and unstable.

Indeed, policy *as* practice is "created" in a trialectic of dominance, resistance and chaos/freedom' (Ball 1994: 11). These dimensions are all to be found in my interviews with the teachers, as they grapple with the immediate effects of the introduction of the 1988 Education Reform Act. Since then other legislation and policies relating to special educational needs have been implemented; they have not been covered here. However, it is hoped that this study contributes to

> our collective understanding of the nature of the complex web of the social forces in which policy-makers, teachers, pupils and other educational professionals and consumers are inextricably enmeshed, and will highlight ways in which different aspects of this intricate reality ultimately impact on the quality of learning, which must remain its fundamental goal.
> (Pollard *et al.* 1994: 4)

Thus the insights that this study provides can be one of 'the many stepping stones in the quest to understand the nature of the educational enterprise and, hence, to provide for it most effectively' (Pollard *et al.* 1994: 4). To achieve its aims, this book is organized into three parts.

Part 1: Setting the theoretical scene

This part is composed of two chapters. Chapter 1 considers the multiplicity of conflicting ideologies and practices that the notion of integration encompasses. Theories of contentious notions such as 'disability', 'normalization' and 'special needs' are analysed in relation to intense discursive struggles to define 'how things are' or 'ought to be'. The aim is to reconstitute the dominant individualistic and medical deficit approach to the above issues both by taking into serious consideration the voices of disabled people and by shifting the focus of analysis onto the complexities and power relationships that are involved in these controversial and wide-ranging debates.

Chapter 2 concentrates on a review of the main findings of previous attitudinal research towards the process of integration. The focus on the existing, mainly conventional, attitudinal research is connected with an attempt to show that the way both attitudes and research have been conceptualized contributes to the perpetuation of a restrictive and often oppressive way of viewing complex issues such as attitudes and disability. A critical analysis of the term 'attitude' is offered which in turn becomes the platform for presenting the fundamental ideological principle underlying the methodological and analytical/interpretative procedures of the present attitudinal study.

Part 2: Teachers' perspectives

Chapter 3 describes the broader educational context as experienced by the teachers who participated in this study. It offers an understanding of how teachers think and feel about their work, and relates this to their professional ideologies and personal priorities. The work context of teachers in a rapidly changing environment is closely interwoven with their attitudes towards the process of integration: a topic which constitutes the theme of Chapter 4.

Chapter 4 explores the way policies made at other levels influence policies in use. It further indicates the ideological/personal constraints within which teachers try to define and implement integration, and the tensions they face in trying to resolve conflicting priorities and contradicting expectations.

Part 3: Children's perspectives

Chapter 5 identifies some crucial issues which are included within the overused and often problematic notion of 'social integration'. The focus is on exploring children's attitudes towards the integration of disabled children, identifying in this way the influence of adult discursive practices on children's emerging ideologies.

Chapter 6 enters into the realm of childhood culture and explores the social and cultural context within which children develop attitudes and ascribe meanings to the complex and often volatile patterning(s) of interpersonal relationships between disabled and non-disabled children. A particular emphasis is placed on the way 'handicapped' identities are socially created.

Finally, even though it is felt that in complex realities, 'research is an exploration, not a finding' (Peters 1995: 70), the book concludes by reconsidering the major themes and offering potential areas for further consideration.

PART 1

SETTING THE THEORETICAL SCENE

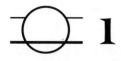 **1**

Disability, normality and special needs: political concepts and controversies

In this book the term 'integration' has a significant role as one of the main concepts under analysis. However, during the search for a working definition of the concept, I realized that such a term encompasses a multiplicity of conflicting ideologies and practices.

The process of defining terms is complex but significant, because definitions serve different, although interdependent, functions; they allow for communication, thought, social interaction and control (see Meighan 1981). That is, on the one hand, they order individuals' personal and social experiences by offering an ideological framework within which people make sense of cultural, social and political phenomena. On the other hand, they are devices for the transmission of these ideological frameworks, including perceptions and conceptualizations, between individuals. Thus, definitions become the means of making sense of the world around us, setting our histories and ideologies in context, and providing a basis for generating action.

From a wider perspective, definitions become even more complicated and significant when they are included in political discourse; within struggles and power relationships they constitute the theoretical basis for attaining an objective. As Fulcher (1989a: 9) argues, 'competing discourses contain a social theory of how . . . the social world works and ought to work'. She goes further by stating that

> Social life may be theorized as consisting of *practical* activities, which are *theoretically* based, and in each of which *social* actors struggle to attain their objectives. This means *practical* activities are simultaneously *theoretical* or *technical*, *moral* and *political*. In other words, discursive practices are theoretically, politically and morally informed.
>
> (Fulcher 1989a: 12, emphasis in original)

Mike Oliver has illustrated the connection between language, definitions and political ideologies by offering reasons why definitions are important. He claims that

> A final reason why definitions are important stems from what might be called 'the politics of minority groups'. From the 1950's onwards there was a growing realization that if particular social problems were going to be alleviated or removed, then nothing more or less than a fundamental redefinition of what the problem actually was, was necessary. Thus homophile groups, black people and women set about challenging the prevailing definitions by attacking the sexist and racist biases in the language used to underpin these dominant definitions and creating, substituting or taking over terminology in order to provide more positive imagery.
>
> (Oliver 1987: 10)

Because of their social function and the involvement of ideology, definitions include an inherent ambiguity and a conflicting multiplicity.

Integration is a social process and its definitions cannot escape from such complexities. It involves a series of parameters with educational, political, moral, theoretical and practical implications. Within the debate of integration a multifaceted divisive discourse has been created which makes it difficult to disentangle rhetoric from institutionalized realities. Pedagogical principles, humanitarian ideologies, theories of normalization, sociopolitical and medical approaches to education are being used in a conflicting way in the cultural struggle of different interest groups; these groups are all trying, within asymmetrical power relationships, to pursue different objectives. Some definitions have a higher degree of 'stickability', to use one of Abberley's (1989) terms, as they are rooted within institutionalized practices and discourses at different levels (see Fulcher 1989a). The degree of stickability of certain discourses is strongly connected to the power some groups hold which enables them to maintain and perpetuate their ideological positions, needs and priorities. Language, knowledge, assumptions, and myths are used to underpin and frame the manifest positions (Atkin 1991).

This chapter is concerned with the ambiguities and conflicting multiplicities inherent in definitions of integration. It is an endeavour to explore the ways the term 'integration' has been used in both the political and practical spheres, and how the ensuing contradictions affect and are affected by other sociopolitical parameters. This chapter attempts to put forward a number of arguments. First, segregation was not mainly about responding to children's needs but rather served and even masked other motives related to society's needs. Second, the preoccupation of defining issues of disability and integration solely from an individualistic medical point of view has further disabled rather than enabled disabled individuals. Such an approach impinges upon efforts for creating inclusive educational systems and has been used to cover the deficiencies of ordinary schools in responding to and educating all children. The issue of normalization is important in such discussion as its definitions are associated with definitions of integration of disabled people in educational and other community settings. Finally, I argue that integration has not been viewed as a commitment to create inclusive education. In addition to this lack of commitment, a number of rhetorical discourses concerning integration have further complicated and obscured what happens in reality.

Segregation: some observations

The debate about implementing integrational policies 'has not taken place in a neutral way but against a cultural and political backdrop of discrimination against disabled people' (Oliver 1987: 9). Understanding Oliver's statement demands an exploration and demystification of the ideologies deployed for the justification of segregation. This is necessary because the term 'integration', first and foremost, implies that the individuals to which it refers have been perceived as different, inferior, and that they have been segregated from mainstream practices.

This differentiation has been based on the principle according to which some children, due to individual deficits, 'cannot cope' within the ordinary educational system. This medical and psychological perspective was further legitimized by a humanitarian ideology that viewed a disabled person as set apart from the rest of society by his/her disability (see, for instance, how a humanitarian religious fervour had pervaded the social perception of disability in nineteenth-century British literature for children (Davidson *et al.* 1994)). Within this context one way of providing for 'the disabled' was to 'protect them from the harsher realities of ordinary school life'. Protection has been synonymous with institutionalization, as these children have had to be educated in special isolated classrooms. Segregated education, however, tends to imply that the children in question have been institutionally destined to live segregated adulthood lives. After all, a 'protective' special educational environment has little in common with the challenges and complexities of an ordinary environment, while 'the result of a "special" education is that children are destined for a "special" life career in terms of employability, self-sufficiency and dependence' (Barton and Tomlinson 1984: 70).

However, humanitarian ideologies have a high degree of stickability because of their connections with notions of 'care', 'love' and 'protection', which are necessary elements within a person's life. Further, Hegel (an early proponent of humanism) 'presented the history of Western civilization as being based on the progressive development of human consciousness' (in Hill 1992: 73). However, it is the same history of humanism, in which institutionalized religions have played a vital role, which has taught us to be suspicious when 'one group claims to be doing good to other groups, particularly when legal coercion is involved' (Tomlinson 1982). While the popular view has been that concern for disabled people has developed as a result of progress, enlightenment and humanitarian interest, 'the experience of this particular group has generally been one of exploitation, exclusion, dehumanization and regulation' (Barton 1986: 276).

Thus the question arises as to what other motives were concealed by humanitarian ideologies. What benefits did the humanitarian aspects of segregation bring to society? Tomlinson (1982), in a sociological analysis of special education, has shown that these motives were related to the wider social and economic interests of a developing industrial society, which required docile bodies and productive people. She indicates that by the early nineteenth-century, education for the mass of the people was regarded as a necessary discipline for controlling potential unrest among the working classes and also for producing a literate population to further commercial interests.

The development of special education was seen as an industry which could produce profits as long as the cost of educating these children could be kept to the minimum. This side of the profit motive was presented as a concern for educating (vocationally training) as many people as possible, which was in agreement with the wider ethic of creating productive citizens that, in turn, would be beneficial for a developing industrial society. Thus the issue which began to emerge was 'how to make as many of the handicapped [sic] productive, while keeping the cost of any provision low so that the central and local government do not have to use too much money provided by non-handicapped [sic] tax- and rate-payers' (Tomlinson 1982: 38).

What, however, was more important within this historical context was the use of education as a means of control and a mechanism for producing obedient and 'moral' citizens. The term 'defective' people was used to identify potentially troublesome and disruptive social groups, mainly originating from the lower working classes, who did not conform to the existing system. Economic and political interest focused on controlling these groups while removing them from the ordinary educational system so as to allow its smooth functioning. Disabled people, especially mentally disabled people and other potentially 'disruptive' groups, were connected, through the influence of the eugenic movement, with crime, immorality, prostitution and unemployment; they were presented as a danger to the smooth functioning of society. As Tomlinson (1982: 40) indicates, 'moves to segregate mentally defective adults and children on account of their possible danger to society very largely contributed to the stigma still attached to special schooling'.

The social history of disability (or 'disabled history' as it has been characterized by Rieser and Mason (1992)) is full of moral discourses of persuasion as to how dangerous disabled people are for society. Morality was, and still is, used as a strong cover for social control mechanisms. For example, Fernald, an influential figure in the area of disability, wrote in 1913:

The feeble-minded are a parasitic predatory class never capable of self support or of managing their own affairs. They cause unutterable sorrow at home and are a menace and danger to the community. Feeble-minded women are almost invariably immoral and if at large usually become carriers of venereal disease or give birth to children who are as defective as themselves . . . Every feeble-minded person, especially the high grade,

is a potential criminal needing only the proper environment and opportunity for the development and expression of his criminal tendencies.

(in Rosen *et al.* 1976: 145)

Also, in 1915, Goddard had written:

> For many generations we have recognized and piled the idiot. Of late we
> have recognized a higher type of defective, the moron, and have discov-
> ered that he is a burden; that he is a menace to society and civilization;
> that he is responsible to a large degree for many, if not all, of our social
> problems.

(in Wolfensberger 1972: 34)

Thus segregation, even though it was presented as a recognition of children's needs and their protection from harsh realities, mainly served other
ends such as economic and political ones (including the need to develop a
social controlling mechanism (Oliver 1985)). However, the popular image of
society protecting its more 'vulnerable' citizens has remained, as it was a good
policy for masking society's contradictions. Translating this to the language
disabled people use in order to understand their position, protectors became
the oppressors and protégés became the oppressed. Within a more modern
society, both charity and lay discourses have been developed prohibiting disabled people from having access to decision-making processes that affect their
lives in the first place. Furthermore, such discourses have located power and
responsibility/interest in the others – the professionals and specialists – by presenting them as those 'best equipped', who have both knowledge of, and
'solutions' to the pathology, and, therefore, power over the person. Power
here is seen as the ability of significant others to define the identity and the
needs of disabled people. The significant other becomes even more powerful
when through legal requirements or voluntarily, s/he undertakes the care of
disabled people imposing simultaneously directly or indirectly a specific status
on them. For instance, Simone Aspis' (1992) personal accounts of the un-
worthy treatment she received during her ten years in a special school are
indicative of the vulnerability of disabled pupils and are illustrative of how she
was made to feel inferior on the basis of the 'others'' definitions of her identity: 'The teachers always told me that I could not achieve anything' (p. 282).

However, the notion of power has been partially disguised by the use of the
notions of concern and interest. As Cole (1989) states, 'special education pio-
neers – and indeed more recent practitioners and policy makers, including
medical officers – generally seemed imbued with a deep concern for the interests of special children' (in Hill 1992: 72).

After a hundred years spent building a complex system of segregation, and
after all the historical and political development of the struggle between
rhetorical discourses of humanitarianism and discourses on the rights of those
called disabled, a new concept has emerged: that of integration. This concept
emerged out of the pressure of some groups – disabled people and advocates
of disabled people's rights – that segregated education is a major cause of

society's widespread prejudices against disabled people. Further, special education 'has always provided something of a dilemma of egalitarianism' (Tomlinson 1982: 46). Within the egalitarian ethic, segregation was perceived as a
violation of basic human rights of disabled people. However, the emerging
concept of integration was, and still is, highly problematic; its analysis reflects
tensions, contradictions and ambiguities which have led some people to
define integration as another name for special education. As Oliver claims,

> Integration as a process has taken on the language of rhetorics; to para-
> phrase Cohen (1985), while the language has changed the same groups
> of professionals are doing the same things to the same groups of children
> as they were before integration was ever mentioned . . . To put the matter
> bluntly, children with special educational needs still get an inferior edu-
> cation to everyone else, and although the rhetorics of integration as a
> process may serve to obscure or mystify this fact the reality remains.
>
> (Oliver 1992b: 23)

The question that arises is, if the movement of integration, as it has been
claimed, rested on the right of disabled children to the same opportunities for
self-fulfilment as other people, then why do disabled children still get an
inferior education to everyone else?

A simple response would be that there were other principles which
informed the integration debate. It could be argued that integration is a cheap
alternative to special education. Throughout the years of building segregated
practices a wide network has developed in which a plethora of specialists and
special equipment have surrounded special schooling. To maintain such a
system could be costly and counter-productive. Thus a good cost-effective
practice, especially in an era of capital crisis, would be to place children with
special educational needs in ordinary education and hide this motive under
the principle of egalitarianism. Local authorities and some teachers base their
scepticism and suspicions with regards to integrational policies and practices
on the above explanation. Even though the issue of cost and resources is
highly significant in promoting integration (and is going to be discussed later
in this chapter), it is not sufficient to explain the complexities involved in the
integration debate. An analysis of these complexities requires first and foremost an exploration of the ways the notion of disability has been defined. The
issue of disability has been perceived differently by different groups of people;
these perspectives are based on certain assumptions and concepts which are
both culturally specific and determined by context.

Defining disability

The predominant point of view perceives disability as a tragic personal affair,
a product of an impairment which is the main cause of disability – even in
cases where clinical factors are not present. This view has been highly influenced by medical discourse on disability, which focuses solely on the clinical

aspects of the human body and pays little attention to its sociopolitical aspects. The language in this discourse uses the notion of disability and impairment synonymously. This medical framework reinforces and is reinforced by charity and lay discourses which define disabled people as 'in need of help (Llewellyn 1983), as an object of pity (Borsay 1986), as personally tragic (Oliver 1986), as 'dependent and eternal children . . . [and] as low achievers by ideal standards' (in Fulcher 1989a: 28). In exploring the dominant way that social institutions respond to people tagged as disabled, Fulcher shows how disability has been constructed as *dependence* through complex procedural politics that aim at greater regulation of the individual: 'Legislation and administrative arrangements construct disability as a *procedurally complex status and experience*, so that disabled people lead unusually tentative lives, which are more than usually contingent on those who hold power in an increasingly contested context' (Fulcher 1989b: 64, emphasis in original).

Such procedures personalize and thus depoliticize issues of disability and provide the basis for 'others', the 'able-bodied/minded', to grant to themselves, unquestionably, the right of taking over the care and the control of the person who has been defined as disabled. The carer obtains a 'liberal' and an 'altruistic' perspective of being there to help, 'forgive' and 'semi-accept'. At the same time this perspective serves the existing distribution of power in institutions and society. The thinking beyond this type of language creates forms that covertly 'justify status, power, and authority' (Apple 1979: 143). Further, the other who is 'in charge and control' psychologically reduces feelings of guilt by projecting a protective, maternalistic or paternalistic attitude towards the 'less fortunate' person.

This deficit approach-rooted within the medical, charity and lay concepts of disability – is central to the way welfare states and educational practices respond to an increasing proportion of citizens (Fulcher 1989a). This is not to say that individual factors should be ignored, for especially where learning is concerned, we cannot reject the existence of factors within the child that inhibit learning; this would be to replace one extreme view with another. As Hegarty (1987: 36) suggested: 'the fact that there is not a direct or invariant link between a given impairment and a particular kind of learning does not mean that there are no links'.

However, such an individualized framework of ability and disability scarcely admits that in educational systems the term 'disability' is being used in such an extraordinarily wide sense; includes not merely impaired-based disabilities but also contentious concepts (i.e. socio-emotionally unstable, disruptive, learning difficulties, learning disabilities, special needs) that conceal 'conflict in social relations and the failure of educational practices' (Fulcher 1989a: 41). An inclusive discourse demands first and foremost an alternative way of 'seeing' and responding to issues of disability.

Disabled theorists, through their struggles, have offered the conceptual means of doing so. Finkelstein (1980: 35), a disabled writer and advocate of an alternative approach to the issue of disability, claims that 'in our view it is society which disables physically impaired people. Disability is something imposed on top of our impairment by the way we are unnecessarily isolated and excluded from full participation in society.'

To understand such a statement, especially if someone has not experienced the oppression that disabled people experience, is not an easy task. This happens for a number of reasons. The predominant medical model has been so powerful that as an ideology it not only shapes consciousness but also has reached into the depths of personality and is being reinforced through the patterns and routines of everyday life. In a sociological analysis of health and illness that attempts to explore what discourses inform the social practices organized around the notion of disability, Fulcher writes that

> The medical model has dominated perceptions of and policy on disability . . . Since society is steeped in the medical model . . ., its professionalism informs the perceptions of a wide range of people. This includes those with formal power (politicians, legislators, administrators), in a wide range of arenas and practices, including social workers, psychologists, rehabilitation counsellors and teachers . . . as well as those with informal, interpersonal power over the lives of people tagged as disabled.
>
> (Fulcher 1989b: 44)

Thus when asking people to express the meaning they attribute to the notion of disability, we must bear in mind that ideology 'as a second nature is history congealed into habit, rooted in the very structure of needs' (Giroux 1984: 317). This implies that the notion of disability has been developed within a wider societal context in which needs and thus priorities are key features.

The predominant understanding of disability as primarily a medical phenomenon reflects, as Fulcher (1989a) has argued, the authority and influence of the medical profession and the extent to which its ideas penetrate and inform everyday and professional discourses on disability. Abberley, in his analysis of the notion of disability as one of oppression, has stated that:

> Definitions with 'stickability' tend to be those produced by groups with power. The most powerful definitions of normality in terms of their effects upon those to whom they are applied are, for disabled people, those propagated and perpetuated by those with the most wide-ranging and immediate power over us, namely the medical and welfare professions.
>
> (Abberley 1989: 57)

Disability is a 'category' constructed by discourses in which the medical ideology has become established due to its powerful position in the hegemony of discourses. According to Huat Chua, 'a discourse is being established as it insinuates itself into the institutionalized arrangements of the social order. It is from these institutional bases that the hegemony of a discourse realizes itself as a practical system of power and a system of social control' (in Fulcher 1989a: 25).

Looking at the history of the development of special needs, and the devaluation of disabled people, Tomlinson (1982: 39) informs us that 'the medical profession struggling for professional recognition in nineteenth-century Britain developed an interest in mental defect, and the profession of medicine was considerably enhanced by medical claims to care for and control the mentally defective'. It was part of a contract between the state, social and economic interests, and the medical profession's interests to segregate and control 'mentally defective' people; bearing in mind that not only disabled but other potentially 'troublesome groups' were identified with that term. This type of contract served a variety of needs which had little to do with disabled people's needs. With regard to the state, economic interests were served by removing 'defective people' who were interrupting workhouse labour, and political interests were served by the confinement of a potentially disruptive social group (see Tomlinson 1982). As far as the medical profession were concerned, such an agreement brought benefits in terms of professional status and economic interest, while educational benefits stemmed from the fact that segregation allowed ordinary schools to proceed more smoothly; which throughout educational history is one of the primary interests of educators. For instance, why do educational and political discourses, when referring to the category of 'socio-emotional difficulties', predominantly focus on 'loud, disruptive and potentially aggressive students' and not on students with quiet withdrawn behaviour? – particularly if we consider that both types of behaviour can impinge upon learning, the enhancement of self-esteem and the development of meaningful relationships within an educational context. As Janet Collins suggests, in an analysis of the way the educational system responds to a group of children defined as 'the silent minority' (i.e. students with a quite withdrawn behaviour, habitually quiet behaviour),

> Evidence from the present study suggests that quiet withdrawn pupils are often overlooked in busy classrooms. Moreover, the fact that few writers include habitually quiet behaviour in their definition of disaffection implies that the term 'emotional and behavioural difficulty' is more likely to be used to define loud, disruptive and potentially aggressive pupils . . . The emphasis on loud potentially disruptive behaviour implies that the concept of special educational need is a form of social control and is used primarily for those pupils who cannot be easily controlled in mainstream classes or who hinder the smooth running of the school.
> (Collins 1994: 152)

The development of these three broadly classified interest groups (state, medical and educational) was not unproblematic, and their relationship included political conflicts stemming out of a concern for protecting and enhancing vested interests (see Tomlinson (1982) for an extensive historical analysis).

The hierarchical medical ordering of the world – even though it is 'conceptually limited and politically limiting' (Fulcher 1989a: 192) – has been strengthened by its advocacy of 'scientific' and ostensibly 'value-free' and apolitical views of what constitutes disability. This world-view provides key rationalizations for the formulation of social practices as natural events (see for instance Abberley's (1992) and Oliver's (1992a) analysis of the OPCS surveys regarding the practices involved in the distribution of disability). In addition, the social connotation of expertise does not allow space for lay people to question and, even harder, to object to professional judgements. The historically powerful domination of a medical discourse 'through its language of body, patient, help, need, cure, rehabilitation and its politics that the doctor knows best, excludes a language of rights . . . [as well as] excludes the theme of the social construction of disability' and its synonyms (Fulcher 1989a: 29).

In an inclusive discourse some demystifications are necessary. First, disability is a *category*; as such it is part of conflicting social relations and has social and institutional conditions of existence, particularly within welfare, health and educational systems (see Hirst and Woolley 1982; Fulcher 1989a). Second, disability is a *disputed category* which has been defined differently by different groups. It is a disputed category because opposing theories exist within discourses. For some, disability is perceived as a tragic personal affair, an individualized deficit which has to be treated and cured (medical, lay and charity discourses); for others it denotes 'need, help and privilege' (Blaxter 1976 and Stone 1984, cited in Fulcher 1989a). For disabled people it is a category of oppression (Oliver 1986; Abberley 1987) and, as such, emphasis must be placed on the importance of the sociopolitical origins of the impairment and the essential social elements that constitute the material bases for ideological phenomena. Finally, for others disability has been used as a procedural category (Fulcher 1989a) and not as something people cannot do. As a procedural category, often the term 'disability' has been used in some discursive practices to justify a greater regulation of the life of a disabled individual, despite the emergence of 'rights' as a central issue in legislation and debate. Thus disability is *'struggled over* in social practices in a range of arenas; . . . it is a political category' (Fulcher 1989a: 24).

The conflicting process of integration is one of the best examples for showing that disability is a politically disputed category. The major conflict derives from the association between the process of integration and the process of normalization, because the principle of normalization is part of the language of the present philosophy of care for disabled people in Britain (Candappa and Burgess 1989). Also, within the notion of integration, there is a fundamental conflicting discourse. At one end of the continuum, the effort is to retain separate traditions but in distinctive departments with their own power bases, leaving them to resolve or harden their differences in an externally unified structure which enables them to coexist and society to believe that they are somehow together (Sayer 1985, 1987). At the other end efforts are made to revise and extend what is seen as the current stage of 'normality' in order to provide for all needs, whether termed 'special', 'vocational', 'life-long' or whatever (Jones 1985; Sayer 1985, 1987). But what constitutes 'normality' and how has this construct been associated with the principle of normalization? Further, how has this principle been defined in theory and in practice, what conflicts does it include, what myths has it produced and how have these myths affected disabled people?

The principle of normalization in theory and in practice

The principle of normalization, the way it has been understood and the manner in which it has been applied in integrational educational practices act upon and reflect the struggles over defining the notion of disability. It has also been used for legitimizing segregation and devaluation for those who do not conform to 'normal' images and standards, and for perpetuating the medical model of disability. It has created a variety of myths which oppress disabled people, depoliticize the issue of disability and bring further confusion and empty rhetoric to impede the establishment of inclusive discourses.

The principle of normalization has been the subject of much debate, confusion and misunderstanding because it includes the construct of 'normality'. Wolfensberger has defined normalization as the 'use of culturally normative means to offer [devalued] persons life conditions at least as good as the average citizens, and to as much as possible enhance or support their behaviour, appearances, experiences, status and reputation' (in Candappa and Burgess 1989: 71).

In expanding this definition Wolfensberger clarified that a person becomes devalued not through his/her 'differentness' itself but through negatively valued 'differentness' which is contingent upon other cultural and social factors. He further suggests that this devaluation can be eliminated by changing the perceptions and values of the perceivers, in which process a necessary condition is to minimize the differentness (stigma) which activates the perceiver's devaluation (in Candappa and Burgess 1989).

The essential issue, and the one which has become the source of confusion, is related to the nature, form and ideologies within the process of 'minimizing difference'. What does this imply? Minimizing the 'difference' according to the normalization principle, in the way it has been defined by Wolfensberger (1972), implies certain actions that change the way society operates. It implies processes of enhancing the cultural stereotype of groups that have been perceived as deviant, in which the representation of disabled people and the allowing of their 'voices' to be heard become a high priority.

This approach necessitates the 'normalization of services' by their physical placement into cultural-typical contexts so as to empower disabled people to have access to every service in the same way as every other citizen does. The assumption behind the normalization of services is that the people putting them into practice perceive the client group as valued. For this to happen there is a need to re-examine staff–client relationships with the aim of de-emphasizing staff–client distinctions. It presupposes relationships which challenge the deeply entrenched ethos of professionalism, by granting to the client equality of knowledge and the right to choose and decide. Consequently, it opposes the ideology that disabled people, and especially mentally disabled people, are incapable of performing functions or making decisions, which staff perform on their behalf (see Candappa and Burgess 1989). Finally, it requires a critical examination of the values and perceptions of the 'carers' who impose domination and devaluation in the name of 'love', 'care' and 'help'. Within this context, the process of normalization is about rights and values; it defines disability as a public highly political affair, in which the state shares responsibility in offering the services needed to respond to its citizens' needs, which indeed are different. It demands exploring the origins and nature of differences and not asserting the normality of disabled people (Abberley 1989). It is a realization that we live in a world of difference and the struggles are for integrating these differences. In a world of difference the concept of normality does not exist. It is a construct that cannot be defined at all.

Within the general population there are those that are deemed 'normal' and those that are perceived as 'deviant'. What is crucial is the realization that the criteria chosen for distinguishing one from the other are socially constructed. It is difficult to find a consensus over the content of these criteria. Through the interaction of the different views of various groups, these criteria are modified, extended and/or altered. What one society perceives as normal another perceives differently.

Further, and crucially importantly, 'within cultural politics, what constitutes normal behaviour depends upon the class status of the protagonists' (Corbett 1991: 260). The way we form our perceptions about what constitutes 'normality' is highly related to our values, orientations, upbringing, needs, priorities and other prior experiences. In addition, those perceptions are highly influenced by the dominant definitions, which are dominant because of their degree of 'stickability'. This, in turn, is related to the power some groups have in institutionalizing the discourse they hold.

In practice, definitions with stickability bear little relevance to the above and have created a number of oppressive practices for disabled people; moreover, their exploration is quite disturbing in a number of ways. In a powerful discussion of the rhetoric versus the reality of the 'human service' policies, Wolfensberger explores the amount and degree of deception inherent in the institutional basis of forming specific definitions based on notions of normalcy and deviancy:

> In the human service field, we are confronted by a great deal of rhetoric, and by an avalanche of documents, that proclaim that services are beneficient, charitable, benign, curative, habilitative, etc. These then are the manifest functions of human service organizations. But while services may be some of these things some of the time, they also commonly perform latent functions very different from these proclaimed ones, including ones that are competency-impairing, destructive of independence, that are actually dependency-making and dependency-keeping.
>
> (Wolfensberger 1989: 26)

In a further substantiating analysis he indicates how and why (according to the latent, as opposed to the manifest, functions of the 'human service supersystem') popular definitions of normalcy and deviancy are formed in such a way as to perpetuate dependency. 'Managing deviancy' and thus defining normalcy, is one among other political processes of responding to our post-primary production patterns of labour that demand such a degree of regulation to the point where 'hardly anybody can do anything for the clients anymore' (Wolfensberger 1989: 34). Because the needs of the clients come last on the agenda of the 'supersystem's' priorities within the process of normalization, the focus has increasingly been on normalizing people.

Further, the medical model used in legitimizing the main functions of such a social system translates the term 'normalization' as 'curing' and 'treating' those characteristics of a person which make him/her different from the majority. This ideology, even though it is being used for further technical progress within medicine, in everyday life can be quite offensive. How, for instance, can a person with Down's Syndrome become a person without Down's Syndrome? It can also be viewed in charity images of disability, such as a poster which presents a wheelchair surrounded by broken chains, saying something like 'break through your chains', in which the physically disabled person who used the chair has disappeared (probably being somewhere else walking?). The caption for the poster declares: 'Volunteer to Help Disabled People Break Free'. The chains are associated with the existence of the wheelchair, which in fact is being used by a physically disabled person as an aid in his/her everyday life activities. The poster implies that it is the impairment – the chair – which chains disabled people, obscuring in this way the barriers and chains that social constructions impose on them. Such posters impose further oppression on disabled people in that they use the wheelchair as an aid to help them with their activities, and therefore they cannot or do not want to 'break free' from it. However, the logic underpinning such charity adverts places disabled people in a stressful and cruel position by forcing them to deny first of all their individual differences (see French 1993). As Morris, a physically disabled writer, claims:

> In our efforts to challenge the medical and the 'personal tragedy' models of disability, we have sometimes tended to deny the personal experience of disability . . . If we deny this we will find that our personal experience of disability will remain an isolated one; we will experience our differences as something peculiar to us as individuals – and we will commonly feel a sense of personal blame and responsibility.
>
> (Morris 1992: 12)

In other cases the principle of normalization has been used in order to indicate that disabled people are normal, not different, and they should be treated equally to everybody else. But the notion of equality here is defined as 'sameness', forgetting that equal does not always mean the same. Abberley has argued that 'During the last 20 years the particular structural changes which have taken place in social work in Britain have had the effect of producing a new but equally damaging "myth" about disabled people, namely that they are "normal"' (Abberley 1989: 59; see also Rowley 1992).

Also, through efforts at 'proving' the normality of disabled people, the focus was transferred from the impairment to the search for other normal conditions of humanity which naturalize disability. Disability was connected with the natural phenomenon of ageing, 'reducing the amount of perceived disability in society, presenting it as "exceptional"' (Abberley 1989: 60), thus imposing additional constraints on young disabled people who have to function in a society within which productivity is a high priority. If we link this with what Morris claimed about the denial of disabled people's experiences then this type of normalization process leads disabled people 'to normalize their situation, thus maintaining the existing structures of social organization and of work' (Abberley 1989: 60). Being forced to deny their difference and normalizing their situation, the working conditions, however, remain the same and become oppressive for them.

What is even more oppressive is the sociopsychological effect of this process on disabled people by the creation of heroic images. Their achievements are being considered as heroic activities handled only by brave people who 'can make it' through the complexities of life. But as Abberley (1989: 62) argues, 'such "heroicism", whilst superficially a more attractive role, is in the long run not an advance for disabled people, since it obscures the social origins of the oppression of disabled people, and encourages the masking of psychological suffering'.

Finally, this external oppression of denying the difference so as to 'be normal' creates another form of oppression for disabled people: internalized oppression. Internalized oppression occurs when a person feels bad about him/herself and wishes to be like someone else. In this case it is also common to feel bad about the group one belongs to and to try to merge her/himself into the group which is perceived as superior in the hope that the difference will become invisible. As Rieser and Mason claim:

> Internalized oppression is not the cause of our mistreatment, it is the result of our mistreatment. It would not exist without the real external oppression that forms the social climate in which we exist. Once oppression has been internalized little force is needed to keep us submissive. We harbour inside ourselves the pain and the memories, the fears and the confusions, the negative self-images and the low expectations, turning them into weapons with which to re-injure ourselves, every day of our lives.
>
> (Rieser and Mason 1992: 27)

This happens not only to disabled people but to other devalued groups such as black people. Research has shown that black children even by the age of 3 were already wanting to be white, as they valued their white friends more than their black friends (research conducted by the Save the Children Fund in Rieser and Mason 1992: 27).

In educational practices the process of normalization – the way it has been viewed and applied – creates a variety of tensions with political implications. Normalization has been viewed as a one-way process in which the focus of attention in most of the practical discourses has been on 'normalizing children'. Children's differences have been characterized as 'special', and integration has been perceived in terms of 'extra' resources and/or children with 'special needs'. Let us examine these issues further.

A critical reflection on the integration process and 'special needs'

It is commonly accepted that some schools offer better provision than others, in the same way as some LEAs have a better record than others on integrating children that were previously segregated (Swann 1985, 1991). However,

> Some historians and social theorists see it as inevitable that schools should create . . . difficulties. Education is a form of social control, designed to fit children into a limited number of life slots, and as universal education spread, it did not respond to children's individual situations. It is unlikely that it could have done even if the intention was there. All children of the same age were assumed to be the same for purposes of instruction, despite the obvious fact that they are not, and given the same educational treatment. Those children who did not fit should have highlighted the inadequacy of the system.
>
> (Hegarty and Pocklington 1981: 37)

Thus children who did not fit into the categories that the educational system has 'so painstakingly allocated for them' (Jupp 1992: 5) became a threat by revealing the system's inadequacies. To cover such inadequacies a variety of mechanisms were developed, according to which the children who 'did not fit' were perceived not as the 'social products' of an insufficient system but as children with 'special needs'; in other words unmet needs were characterized as 'special needs'. The Warnock Report *Special Educational Needs* (1978) is central to any discussion of the complexities involved in the use of this term.

Mary Warnock (1991) interpreted this concept as a move away from the medical model based on diagnosis of defects, which was the source of previous categorizations of children after their impairment. This happened because, as Jupp (1992: 5) has indicated, 'it has become obvious to many who are currently employed within human services, as it has to many who use these services, that whenever we insist upon drawing such arbitrary lines and planning in this way, there will always be those who do not fit into the categories we allocated for them'. It was also a result of the struggles to avoid categorizing people by using offensive labels.

The introduction of the term 'special needs' was supposed to be wider and more general as there was a need to find a term which would include the increasing numbers of children (18 to 20 per cent) who were characterized as having learning or other difficulties. Due to its ambiguity and vagueness it was also supposed to have positive rather than negative overtones. The first point to be made, however, is that the introduction of this term was anything but a move away from the medical way of thinking, according to which 'needs' are deficit-based 'with an inbuilt tendency to slip back towards individuals and their problems' (Collins 1994: 173).

The term implies that 'a child has a learning difficulty if he or she has a significantly greater difficulty in learning than the majority of children of his or her age. Presumably, all such children require some special education provision and all, therefore, must be regarded as having special educational needs' (Hegarty 1988: 43). The first anomaly originates from the way this term has been associated with acquiring provision through statementing procedures. The within-the-child difficulties have been used to legitimize 'extra-special provision'. In order to provide 'extra provision', the child's needs have to be legitimized as deficiencies. Second, to use 'needs statements' as a sufficient basis for developing policy and practice is to ignore that 'to be entitled to something is very different and more positive than to need it, since it gives both validity and value to the claim' (Roaf and Bines 1989: 15). Third, to need 'extra provision' is a clue that education is not constructed to include all children. Education is actually designed to include some children, with subsequent efforts and struggles to broaden provision for those who do not fit in. Thus to cover the deficiency of educational provision children's needs have to be looked at, institutionalized, legitimized and, furthermore, cured and normalized. Integration is here presented as being about children with 'special needs'. But in this case, as Barton and Oliver (1992: 14) maintain, 'by emphasizing the pupil's failure the fundamental issue of the system's failure to meet needs of all pupils is masked'.

Furthermore, the introduction of this vague term and its ensuing practical problems has created a number of complexities and contradictions. The term is so broad, vague and relative that it takes on different meanings according to the context in which it is used (usually based on professional and value-judgements); it also refers to children with a wide range of strengths and weaknesses. As Collins indicates,

> The problem with 'needs', as currently understood, is that it is a term which often serves to mask category and disadvantage without actually specifying or overcoming these in any way . . . 'Needs' has become a category as in 'special needs children', gathering together widely different groups who are then assumed to be defective in some way.
>
> (Collins 1994: 177)

This term encourages the perception of children as a homogeneous group, focusing on their 'commonality' of being 'special'. The term 'special needs', throughout its extensive use within discourses at different levels (i.e. bureaucratic, legislative, educational, administrative and so on), has been used to refer to children who have or may not have an impairment. Thus there has been a conflation of 'normative and non-normative categories of handicap' (Tomlinson 1982; Barton and Tomlinson 1984). The term 'special needs' has been ultimately defined as disability even in cases where an impairment is not present. This is a highly political act as it further reduces the exploration of the social context of learning. From this perspective integration is presented as being about children with disabilities.

The introduction of such a vague term facilitates the projection of inconsistencies implicit in policy-making. The same term employed in political discourses of integration and characterized by Warnock as having positive connotations, in practice has been used to perpetuate exclusive education, difference and inferiority. As Tomlinson highlights,

> The Warnock recommendations and the government approach do go some way towards accommodating egalitarian critics of segregation, while keeping what counts as 'special needs' as vague as possible in order to accommodate segregation where it is deemed necessary. Functional integration, for example, could still ensure that a child is being removed from his or her normal classroom and tagged with the label 'special' which carries a historical stigma of difference and inferiority.
>
> (Tomlinson 1982: 78)

Going further, the 1981 Education Act (which was based on the recommendation of the Warnock Committee) indicates that:

> Where a local authority arranges special education provision for a child . . . it is their duty to provide [this] in an ordinary school [provided that] account has been taken of the views of the child's parents and *is compatible with*:
> (a) his receiving the special educational provision that s/he requires,
> (b) the provision of efficient education for the children with whom s/he will be educated and,
> (c) the efficient use of resources.
>
> (quoted in CHM 1982: 6–7)

In other words, a child defined as having 'special needs' can be excluded from ordinary education if resources deemed necessary are, for a number of reasons, not in place. In this way, with regards to the majority of children in the mainstream, the vague term of 'special needs' indicates a transference of features of the school environment into something that the child possesses (Hegarty and Pocklington 1981). Thus integration is here presented as being about resources and/or being simply a technical issue to be achieved through the deployment of special equipment and 'special' personnel to ordinary schools. This view sees the economy as providing the principles which would shape educational practice (Fulcher 1989a). Economic interest always lies beyond discourses about resources and provision. As Tomlinson (1982: 57) indicates, economic interests, however, dictate that there will be no widespread 'integration' of children who are currently assessed out of the normal system back into it, for as one commentator has noted: 'the three words that appear most often in the White Paper . . . are not . . . special educational needs, they are Present Economic Circumstances'.

The issue of resources has been a never-ending cause of contention within the integration debate. Tony Hercock's (Rotherham's assistant director of services) response when asked about the progress of integration was: 'We had a very strong special schools base before the 1981 Act and would have been foolish to dismantle it over a night ['over a night' being defined as a time-duration of ten years]. The easy and cheaper option would have been to close some of our special schools as has happened elsewhere. But you cannot do that and guarantee continued support' (Hercock 1991).

In an era of capital crisis, notions of practicability, efficiency and cost are very important and can be heard quite often when the issue of integration arises. On the one hand, the supposed aim of these three conditions is to ensure a high quality of 'special' educational provision, including physical organization of facilities and expertise of the teaching staff. On the other hand it includes 'the avoidance of unreasonable expenditure'. The term 'un-reasonable' is relative and subject to various interpretations, according to the priorities of government representatives. Educational provision for children with special educational needs is the last challenge on the list of political priorities and, in conjunction with the social devaluation of disabled people, it tends to be the first area to suffer from financial cuts imposed on education. In an era of economic constraints, an integration debate which focuses solely on resources and cost-effectiveness contains the danger of integration being viewed as a cheap alternative to special education. As Roger Slee's (1993) analysis of the politics of integration reminds us, the debate about resourcing integration seems to have been blighted by a form of reductionism even though the deployment of resources is an important aspect for the creation of inclusive education.

Furthermore, provision for children with special educational needs has always been identified as 'extra resources', which are specifically provided for the children in question. This view of the within-the-child 'special' needs – which is dominant in practical discourses, and partially originates from the focus on (or lack of) resources – can clarify Warnock's statement that 'special needs' are *relevant*. However, despite mentioning that needs are relevant to the social context in which they are developed (Warnock 1978: 37), the report failed to act on its analysis and use the issue of integration as a means for creating more inclusive educational practices.

In contrast, its perpetuation of the division between ordinary and special provision maintained and even magnified the division between 'ordinary' and 'special' children. In practice this contradiction has become the basis of the creation of a new 'language of handicap' (i.e. the resource children, the inte-grated child). Also the perpetuation of linking educational provision with resources and cost-effectiveness inhibited the Warnock Committee from being committed to an analysis of other aspects of educational provision such as curriculum content, and from exploring the principles which inform decisions about the type and nature of knowledge provided to children. Thus the report has been criticized for failing to link integration to reforms of com-prehensive primary and secondary schooling and the forms of organization, teaching and curricula that are required in the 'integrated' school (Booth 1981). In other words, it has been criticized for divorcing the integration of

children with special educational needs from those policies which significantly affect the comprehensive education of all children (Quicke 1981).

The Warnock Report has also been criticized for perpetuating and strengthening professionalism. A discourse of provision from the perspective of
resources 'is part of professionalism since expertise implies additional costs'
(Fulcher 1989a: 51). This is manifested in the inconsistency included in the
report, which both advocated a continuum response while perpetuating separate services and heightened specialism (Sayer 1987). There are a number
of important issues which can be raised about the increased educational
involvement and powers of professionals in deciding which children do have
special educational needs and their educational placement.

Within the lobby of professionals, teachers have historically been defined
as a low-status occupational group, compared for instance to the medical profession. This is partly due to the perception that they do not hold any expert,
superior knowledge and partly to the variety of criticism of their professional
functioning. They do not posses this type of 'expertise' that could enable them
to create an aura of mystery around their work; it was more difficult for them
to legitimize procedures of identifying children as having 'special needs'. Due
to this lack of expertise, ordinary teachers were not perceived as adequate in
teaching these children, as it was considered that 'special needs' demanded
special teachers.

The creation of this new interest group called 'special teachers' was initially accepted and even promoted by ordinary teachers, as benefits derived for
them out of such 'bargaining'. This can be illustrated by a comment from a
special school head teacher who wrote:

> Special school teachers were felt to have left the main field of education
> and were looked on as missionaries going into an unknown field . . .
> teachers in ordinary schools were glad that some of their profession had
> elected to do what they felt was distasteful . . . cope with defective chil-
> dren.
>
> (Lindsay 1951, cited in Tomlinson 1982: 91)

Thus being a special teacher was surrounded by a social context which actually devalued the concept of being 'special'. This derived from the perceived
nature of educating children who were viewed as inferior and more difficult
to teach. However, special teachers benefited as well through the development of a specialized network. They became specialists; the specialism
was legitimized and further institutionalized within higher education by the
preparation and qualifying of teachers who would have to work in a whole
new area, special education. Thus a divisive institutionalized policy was developed which reinforced the distinction of educating some teachers to become
special and some to become mainstream.

The new group developed vested interests and became involved in struggles
of protecting (and enhancing) the benefits derived from their occupational
involvement with their new clientele. The well-established view was – and
still is – that special teachers are necessary for some children and 'this view

suggests or articulates a particular range of objectives for special education, such as: identifying "difference", separate career structures, a focus on dis-ability and so on' (Fulcher 1989a: 9).

In the same way as resources, specialism has become another prominent controversy within the integration debate. The dominant focus is on the acquisition of 'special' skills, and it has created the view that ordinary teachers have to acquire such skills in order to teach children with special educational needs. As Fulcher argues,

> The institutional bases for the educational version of a discourse on deficits, difference and professionalism, which lie in teaching training institutions which separate skills for teaching those deemed disabled, were reinforced: there was to be in-service training for regular teachers to gain necessary expertise.
>
> (Fulcher 1989a: 165)

Thus the first divisive practices originate out of the splitting of relationships, roles and responsibilities between two types of teachers – 'special' and 'ordi-nary' – who are both teaching the same class (a point further analysed in the discussion of the results of this study).

Galloway and Goodwin's (1987) and Fulcher's (1989a) view that teachers have become key policy-makers in regard to exclusive or inclusive practices is crucial. The inconsistencies of the legislation have offered teachers the opportunity to interpret the law in different ways according to different pur-poses, allowing them – if they are not committed to inclusive education – to have the power of excluding children from ordinary schools. As Booth (1983) notes, the overwhelming conclusion is that where integration does not happen it is because people with the power to make the changes do not want children with disabilities in our schools.

To claim, however, that teachers hold such a degree of power that they determine policies is somehow naive and unfair towards teachers – especially if we consider the structural constraints within which they have to work. It is more the case that teachers are being influenced and are influencing inte-grational policies made at other levels. Also the essential point here is that a conflict has developed between the egalitarian ideology of integrating all chil-dren in the same schools, and the need to separate out all children who may be troublesome (in the widest possible sense). This conflict is inherent in both the Warnock Report and the 1981 Education Act, which were perceived as having an impact on changing terminologies, forms and ideologies, yet in reality perpetuated the same underlying infrastructures and purposes of seg-regation, this time within ordinary schools (Tomlinson 1982; Swann 1985; Fulcher 1989a; Oliver 1992b). Also it is essential to note that both documents projected a lack of commitment to define integration as the educational apparatus's failure to provide an inclusive education (a point further discussed later in this chapter).

Jupp illustrates this in a vivid way:

The Warnock report which came and went more than ten years ago now
. . . in practice seemed to have had a minimal effect. The 1981 Education
Act followed; it was born very weak, it died and was then buried without
a proper funeral or even an obituary. They both seem to have been forgotten and are now being pushed aside, in today's scramble to implement
the National Curriculum, Local Financial Management and a host of
other newly acquired responsibilities.

(Jupp 1992: 7)

Overall, the weak commitment of the political discourse/rhetoric towards
inclusive education (see Evans *et al.*'s 1990 analysis of the implementation of
the 1981 Education Act) and the lack of serious consideration of disabled
people's rights, followed by a preoccupation with costs, specialism, professionalism and so on, led to the perpetuation of a strong discourse focusing on
the issue of disability rather than the way(s) schools are functioning. Furthermore the needs that were prioritized had very little to do with the needs of
the so-called 'disabled' or 'special children'. The lack of commitment to
respond to children's needs becomes even more evident in an analysis of the
priorities asserted by the new trend in education.

A new ethos for education

The English and Welsh education system is in the middle of a dramatic period
of transformation in which patterns of access, forms of control and the
nature of the curriculum have all been subjected to change. Even though
there is a conflict of feelings towards the nature of the consequences stemming from the introduction of the 1988 Education Reform Act, there seems
to be an agreement among commentators that it has had a major impact on
the governance, structure, content and outcomes of schooling (Brehony
1990; Kelly 1990; Murphy 1990; Stillman 1990; Abbot and Croll 1991;
Barton and Oliver 1992; Pollard 1992). Barton and Oliver's (1992: 17)
examination of the Educational Reform Act and its relation to integration
argues that 'we are in the midst of an extensive restructuring of educational
provision and practice'.

The introduction of the 1988 Act was both a result of and a stimulus to a
programme of increased economic competition that requires national standards and skilled citizens. It includes a marketing ideology whereby (according to the representatives of the government), consumers (ostensibly
children, whose absence from most contemporary discussions of consumer
choice is interesting in itself, and parents) are granted the capacity to choose
and acquire control over the schools. The passing of the Act was claimed to
increase the autonomy of schools and their responsiveness to parental choice
(DES 1987a). Choice and accountability were presented as key concepts of
the new educational philosophy, accompanied by rhetoric concerned with
'raising standards' generally. Thus it was thought that standards and choice
would be extended by:

- introducing a local financial management scheme that provides the framework for a system of voucher-based funding for schools (Thomas 1990);
- allowing schools to opt out (GM schools) and be directly financed from the central government;
- stating national educational standards, attainment targets, programmes of study;
- introducing a common National Curriculum and presenting it as a yardstick for 'equal' treatment for all pupils (though it is highly disputable how 'equal' a curriculum can be when the consequences of other accompanying measures all conspire to deny it having any meaningful effect on an egalitarian approach to the education of all children (Whitty 1990: 21–35));
- making explicit the goals children are to pursue, the curriculum followed and the learning levels which have been achieved in comparison to national targets;
- implementing standardized national assessment tests;
- requiring schools to publicize their examination results; and
- framing the role, constitution and membership of schools' governing bodies; thus consumers would be informed of the functioning of their school and could choose accordingly.

It has been claimed that by offering opportunities for schools to become self-managed and/or more autonomous, the distribution of resources will become a subject of public debate in which parents will voice their concerns and oppositions. Further, by pressurizing schools and making them accountable to their consumers, a marketing competition will take place among schools, and this will consequently reinforce standards of learning and teaching, particularly as the funding of schools is related directly to the number of pupils on roll. Thus the government has extensively intervened in education in their drive to introduce a competitive market system for the supply of educational services.

A marketing language has emerged which entered the world of education: we have expressions such as delivery of the goods, competition, competitors, offer and demand, cost-effectiveness, providers, clients or consumers, users of the system, and senior management teams. Bearing in mind that language is both a sensitive indicator and a powerful creator of the underlying ideologies and assumptions inherent within political discourses (Apple 1979), it is evident that education is being perceived as a part of a marketing system, as a national investment. For instance, while historically HMI (one of the most powerful groups of professional educationalists) were required to have had considerable teaching experience – usually in senior positions in schools – recently there were indications that this requirement is changing. Powell and Solity (1990: 15) inform us that an advert for HMI which appeared in *The Times Educational Supplement* on 12 May 1989 stated: 'applicants are usually aged between 35 and 45 with experience drawn from successful careers in education but also increasingly, from commerce and industry'.

As Kelly (1990: 48) notes, the picture is that of a factory-farming approach to schooling; he quotes Elliot Eisner (1985), who has summed this up in his description of the 'job analysis' approach to educational planning which began to be favoured in the early part of this century:

> The school was seen as a *plant*. The superintendent directed the operation of the plant. The teachers were engaged in a job of *engineering*, and the pupils were the *raw material* to be processed in that plant according to the demands of the consumers. Furthermore, the product was to be judged at regular intervals along the production line using *quality control standards* which were to be quantified to reduce the likelihood of error. *Product specifications* were to be prescribed before the raw material was processed. In this way efficiency, measured with respect to cost primarily, could be determined.
>
> (Eisner 1985, in Kelly 1990: 48, emphasis in original)

Within the history of education there is evidence that schoolchildren are the least powerful interest group in influencing or participating in decision processes which affect their lives. As Blishen (1969: 67) stated, 'in all the millions of words that are written annually about education, one viewpoint is invariably absent, that of the child, the client of the school. It is difficult to think of another sphere of social activity in which the opinions of the consumer are so persistently overlooked.'

In the document published by the Department of Education and Science (DES) and the Welsh Office in July 1987 entitled *The National Curriculum 5–6: A Consultation Document*, it was declared that the National Curriculum will 'enable schools to be more accountable for the education they offer to their pupils, individually and collectively' (DES 1987b: 4–5). Some lines further it was declared that 'Employers, too will have a better idea of what a school leaver will have studied and learnt at school irrespective of where s/he went to school' (p. 5). In a highly competitive society within which the supply of labour far outstrips demand, the intention is that employers and not children influence the nature of the curriculum, its philosophy, structure, funding and control. As Powell and Solity (1990: 6) indicate, 'The Secretary of State has been determined to ensure that the local community, especially the business community, shall have its views represented to the school.' Further, Kelly (1990), in a critical analysis of the ideologies underpinning the new educational policies, argues that if teachers resort to commercial competitiveness hidden within the new political rhetoric, children can only be the losers. This is partly because what is being offered to children is a 'common curriculum' which imposes on all of them the values of its creators. It can be argued that 'every aspect of every curriculum is value-laden – the choice of subjects, the choice of content, the choice of aims, the choice of models and approaches. And those values are communicated to the recipients of that curriculum in very subtle ways' (Kelly 1990: 99). A highly centralized curriculum (a) perceives teachers mainly as 'the service deliverers', (b) circumscribes significantly their professional autonomy (Pollard 1990), and (c) has been designed with little reference to previous research in regard to children's social world and to the influence of their different sociocultural backgrounds on their learning. Such a curriculum and its practices create an alien and alienating culture for some children, by imposing a set of values which may be in conflict with their own, with all the resulting consequences. Such an imposition is more significant because 'the principles underpinning the legislation are very different from the social-democratic, egalitarian and child-centred ideas to which most primary school teachers have subscribed in the past' (Pollard 1990: 74).

The question that arises now is where does the inclusion of children with special educational needs stand within such a context, and how will it be affected by these new values and priorities? Inclusive education seems to be incompatible with a system that has highly prioritized mechanisms of assessment, sameness, commercialism, elitism, productiveness and notions of effectiveness derived from its economic-industrialized perspective. According to Barton and Oliver,

> Centralized control is being accomplished through the articulation of a new vision over what schools must achieve and how that success and effectiveness is to be defined and monitored. Central to this approach is a belief in the importance of competition and consumer choice . . . Within this climate pupils with special educational needs are not viewed as politically significant and questions of social justice and equity become marginalized.
>
> (Barton and Oliver 1992: 17)

They go further, by stating that, 'The possibility of establishing a comprehensive integration policy becomes more difficult. Indeed, the whole question of integration may well become an increasingly contentious issue' (p. 17). On the other hand, in *Curriculum Guidance: The National Curriculum and Pupils with Severe Learning Difficulties* (NCC 1992: 3), it has been clarified that

> The principle that all pupils should receive a broad and balanced curriculum, relevant to their individual needs is now for the first time established in law. For pupils with special educational needs this entitlement represents an opportunity to improve standards further, building on the advances of recent years as highlighted in the Warnock Report and the 1981 Act (Circular number 5, NCC 1989).

Such a statement does not give reassurance that disabled children will have access to enabling educational opportunities within ordinary education. In contrast, the philosophy underpinning the new policies in regard to the context, form, structure, and implementation of the curriculum excludes any serious consideration of inclusive education.

The political and economic directives surrounding the notions of progress, and the values included in the particular image of the 'normal child', widens the gap between ability and 'disability' by culturally overestimating ability. It strengthens the perception of the individual as an achiever or a failure and gives stronger emphasis to the cognitive function of the individual. The focus on the within-the-child difficulties or 'incapabilities' might be strengthened in order to contribute to explaining why some children fail in a system that provides 'a legal entitlement of all pupils to a broad and balanced curriculum'. As Russell (1990: 215) notes, 'many of us are already cynical about the emphasis given to disability even within schools which have an "equal opportunities" policy'.

Even though individual teachers differ about the nature of their own aims and the way they respond to the immense ideological/educational changes that they are confronted with; and even though they still have the power of the 'face to face action' with children, it is important to bear in mind that teachers 'have, in a sense been "caught in a trap", torn between the aims which they espouse and the means to bring them about' (Pollard 1990: 70). For instance, even teachers committed to inclusive education may find themselves constrained in responding effectively to the challenges posed by children with special educational needs, because of the increasing pressures of 'raising the standards' of their school.

The intensification of competitiveness can make the commitment to inclusive education difficult to maintain. If we look at all the increasingly various and often contradictory demands facing teachers and schools (Blyth 1990), accompanied by strategies required for coping with the logistics of manageability (Dearing 1994), such a commitment becomes even more onerous.

Thus there is an urgent demand for struggles over inclusive education to be intensified by attacking the core of the problem – the curriculum and the values underpinning it. It is via the curriculum (in its context, content, form, structure, and implementation) that policies exercise control by imposing certain ideologies, values, needs and priorities. As Fulcher (1989a: 54) has already argued, 'Since integration is about discipline and control rather than disability, it is at the centre rather than the periphery of educational practices. It may therefore be argued that it is the *educational apparatus's failure to provide an inclusive curriculum*, rather than the problems specific "disabilities" pose, which constructs the *"problems and the politics of integration"* ' (emphasis in original).

From this perspective, integration is about the way ordinary schools are functioning; their effectiveness has to be analysed in terms of how successful or not they have been in integrating differences. Central to this approach is the perception of the curriculum not only as a device for transferring knowledge and acquiring skills but as a means of transferring values to individuals (children) who rely heavily on an adult's constructed world. This involves teachers critically reflecting upon the values they are transferring and the ways they are doing so in their everyday practices. In turn,

Some understanding of the dilemmas, transient as well as deep-seated with which teachers are confronted, is a necessary step towards effective action, both by teachers themselves and by those outside the profession who are genuinely and influentially concerned about what goes on in primary education.

(Blyth 1990: 191–2)

Conclusion

In this chapter I have argued that the notion of integration does not share a common meaning among different groups of people and does not have a single definition. It has more than one meaning in that it reflects the experiences, practices, ideologies and interests of particular groups that interact within asymmetrical power relationships. I have tried to show how a written policy can be internally inconsistent, indeed that its theoretical positions can be antithetical. As Fulcher maintains,

> This reveals the struggles in the policy-writing process, struggles which occur despite a report being presented as consensus. These 'inconsistencies' in policy are often articulated in policy analysis as 'tensions' between principles, but in a political concept of policy they are more accurately seen as the outcome of struggles between parties contending to achieve their different objectives.
>
> (Fulcher 1989a: 7)

Further, it has been noted that within the process of integration, characterizing some needs as 'special' denotes that ideas arising from the practices of special education have been imposed on the integration process, limiting visions of educational opportunity for all. The loose definition of 'special needs' and the way it has been used within different educational structures are mechanisms that perpetuate segregated ideologies even within integrated settings. It has been indicated that, on the one hand, the maintenance and perpetuation of such differentiation promote the retention of traditional notions of 'handicap' and, in turn, demand the retention and extension of those factors which characterize special schooling. On the other hand, they strengthen the focus on pupils for justifying failure. Individualizing – and thus decontextualizing – the creation of learning difficulties conceals the inefficiencies of an educational system that has been constructed to include some children and not others.

This divisive ideology within political discourses, between 'special' and 'ordinary' needs – which has been translated to a division between 'special' and 'ordinary' children – derives partially from a lack of commitment to inclusive education. In conjunction with the new trends emphasizing regulation and market forces (competition, open enrolment) it reflects a lack of serious thought about the right of all children to be included in ordinary schools. It has been argued that, within the current climate, children with special educational needs can become more vulnerable because individual differences are perceived as deficits that impinge upon the smooth functioning of 'raising standards' within ordinary schools.

However, within the struggle of defining integration, an alternative approach has emerged, mainly through the efforts of pressure groups (disabled people) and advocates of inclusive education, according to which both integration and attitudes towards integration should be explored from the analysis of the social environment and its responses towards differences. Such an analysis problematizes the already existing linguistic system that perpetuates unequal relationships, examines the role and the relationships between professionals and disabled people, and explores the new educational trends in regard to their relationship and impact upon integration policies and practices. Such an exploration can indicate the effect of political discourses, made at other levels, on everyday educational practices. It also enables us to identify those institutionalized processes (actions) and ideologies that perpetuate exclusive practices. The principle underlying the examination of attitudes that this study is based on supports Finkelstein's argument, according to which

> The predominant focus of attitudes, help, research and so on, has as a neutral expression of one side of the disability relationship, been towards the disabled person. Nearly all references concerned with attitudes towards disability use the disabled person as the point of focus. The emergent approach is to focus on the behaviour, roles, perceptions, attitudes etc. of the helpers as representatives of a socially determined relationship.
>
> (in Oliver 1987: 10)

However, the nature and complexity of the construct 'attitudes' make the exploration of those attitudes a difficult affair. It has become even more difficult to explore attitudes because of a dominant perception that attitudes are abstract ideologies located in the sphere of the unconscious and revealed differently in different situations.

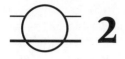 **2**

Towards a better understanding of attitudes

Existing attitudinal research has approached the analysis of integration from a variety of interdependent perspectives. The first includes the effects of labelling on attitudes, and stigma attachment to disabled children in educational settings (Gottlieb 1974; MacMillan *et al.* 1974; Kurtz *et al.* 1977; Siperstein *et al.* 1980; Bromfield *et al.* 1986; Eayrs *et al.* 1993). A second set of studies investigated the social adjustment of disabled people in integrated settings by measuring their self-concept and their sociometric status, comparing it with the self-concept and status of children being in segregated settings (Cassidy and Stanton 1959; Thurston 1959; Mayrowitz 1962; Carroll 1967). A third group of studies measured/explored peers' attitudes towards and interactions with disabled children (Baldwin 1958; Jordan 1959; Goodman *et al.* 1972; Sheare 1974; Cavallero and Porter 1980; Hoben 1980; McHale and Simeonsson 1980; Rynders *et al.* 1980; Johnson and Johnson 1981; Kennedy and Thurman 1982; Sanberg 1982; Miller and Gibbs 1984; Bak and Siperstein 1986; Lynas 1986; Karagiannis 1988; Lewis and Lewis 1988; Shapiro and Morgolis 1988; Siperstein *et al.* 1988; Bowman 1989; Jenkins *et al.* 1989; Kyle and Davies 1991). Finally, there are others which focused on teachers' attitudes and factors influencing the formation of their attitudes (Baker and Gottlieb 1980; Hegarty and Pocklington 1981; Reynolds *et al.* 1982; Aloia and MacMillan 1983; Leyser and Abrams 1983; Stainback *et al.* 1984; Feldman and Altman 1985; Thomas 1985; Bowman 1989; Pinhas and Schmelkin 1989; Clough and Lindsay 1991).

Different studies involve different views of 'integration' and mainstreaming, including different assumptions, processes and implications. Also, as indicated in Chapter 1, progressive policies for promoting integration have not been the official view, and often policies impinge upon practices and vice versa. Thus it was expected that attitudinal research regarding integration would reveal conflicting feelings and opinions, reflecting the different views in the wider social spectrum (Quicke *et al.* 1990). Based mainly on thematic categorization, the following discussion will concentrate on a review of the main findings of the above studies. This review has a two-fold purpose. First, it sheds light on how the process of integration has been tackled, what has been done and what previous researchers have found. Second, the majority of the following analysis will act as a platform for a further consideration and reconstruction of the way the issues of integration and attitudes have been approached by previous conventional attitudinal research.

Attitudes towards integration and the process of labelling

Theories of deviance and labelling have strong historical roots. They were originally developed by sociologists in the study of crime and have since been applied to disabled people (Eayrs *et al.* 1993). In the area of integration a number of arguments have been produced for and against the use of labels, causing considerable controversy. There are circumstances (defined by the 1981 Education Act) in which some labels have been abandoned (i.e. 'educationally subnormal'), being replaced with other labels ('severe or moderate difficulties'), based on the assumption that the latter terms have a more positive connotation than the former.

Other authors claimed that the term 'label' itself has both a specific and a general use. According to Eayrs *et al.* (1993) the first use is connected with unequal relationships in which powerful groups have the means and are able to define the way less powerful groups are perceived and treated. The second is a more commonplace usage in a looser sense, where a term is used to describe another person.

Disabled people and advocates of the rights of disabled people insist on abandoning labels altogether and focus more on the person and his/her social experiences. Oliver (1992b) strongly advocates that going back and examining what able-bodied theorists and researchers have maintained 'is not very useful in understanding the real nature of disability or indeed, integration in modern society . . . If disability is socially created . . . then such arguments are both sterile and futile' (pp. 20–2). He further claims that 'A start can be made by not talking over our heads about issues that are irrelevant to our needs and by allowing us the dignity of deciding what we want to be called' (p. 26).

Oliver (1992b) believes that the way to deal with disablist societies is to change what people do, not what people think. But ways of thinking highly influence ways of living and doing, and one cannot be detached from the other. If this is the case, then the information we have been offered about the effects of labelling on able-bodied attitudes towards disabled people, directly or indirectly is going to affect our actions. To 'join the struggle' of disabled people against a disablist society means first of all to internalize, as an able-bodied person, that society is disablist. One way of reaching this state is to go through the history of information offered by research and critically reflect upon it. A review of empirical studies regarding the use and effects of labelling shows that the issue is highly complicated, with conflicting feelings and opinions.

MacMillan *et al.* (1974) identified five areas in which labelling could affect disabled children: self-concept, peers' rejection, future vocational adjustment, family attitudes and teachers' expectations. After reviewing the available literature in each of these areas, they concluded that there was little support for the notion that disabled children were stigmatized by being labelled as 'retarded'. Gottlieb (1974), examining whether the label 'mentally retarded' influenced peers' attitudes towards disabled people, found that middle-class children are influenced more by the level of academic competence they witness in a child than by the label attached to the child. He interpreted this finding to mean that labels do not lead to negative attitudes that are associated with stigma.

Gottlieb (1986) went further by pinpointing that children's observable behaviour could stigmatize them in the eyes of their peers, regardless of whether they are formally labelled by the school as being 'retarded'. He also claimed that if this is the case and children's inappropriate behaviour contributes to their social rejection by peers, then integrating them into ordinary schools could result in greater ostracism than if they were educated in segregated classes. He justified this argument on the basis that children's inappropriate behaviour will be more visible in an ordinary school.

As far as the effect of labelling on teachers' attitudes is concerned, Kurtz *et al.*'s (1977) study, which used both experimental (labelled) and control (non-labelled) children, found that the label did produce a biasing effect, but in this case the effect was positive. They found that rather than responding negatively to the label, teachers responded in a positive manner by showing less social distance. Their finding was in agreement with Siperstein *et al.* (1980), Towne and Joiner (1968), and also Goodman *et al.* (1972) as cited in the literature review of Gottlieb's (1974) study. These three studies found that labelling may have a protective effect; they have even pointed out potential benefits. For instance, by using an adjective checklist attitude scale, Siperstein *et al.* (1980) found that the label 'mentally retarded' has a beneficial effect as it offers 'a reason' to peers for explaining and understanding their disabled peer's academic incompetence or 'inadequate' behaviour. The authors of this study argued that if no explanations had been given then children may proceed to make unfavourable comparisons between themselves and their disabled peers.

In contrast, Bromfield *et al.* (1986) found that labelling has an influence but not a positive one. They claimed that labelling has a negative effect because teachers have low expectations of their pupils resulting from labelling; consequently the children are likely to underachieve. This experimental study, conducted by the use of video-tapes and questionnaires, revealed that the participants who were presented with a 'mentally retarded' label for the child in the video were less likely to attribute the child's failure to low effort or to environmental factors.

Dandy and Callen (1988) stated that there are a number of other studies using both attitudes and observed behaviour as measures and they tend to show an effect of labelling, although not a strongly consistent one. They also

claimed that showing that there is a labelling effect does not tell us if alternative terms used in integrated settings such as 'learning difficulties' or 'having
special educational need' are more or less influential than the old categories.

A more recent study by Eayrs *et al.* (1993) investigated the effect of three
different labels in current usage on public perceptions of the groups so
labelled. The labels contrasted were 'mentally subnormal', 'mentally handicapped' and 'people with learning difficulties'. Three independent groups of
subjects were presented with an attitude questionnaire. The main findings of
this study supported the view that the term 'learning difficulties' is associated
with more positive attitudes than either of the other labels, whose results do
not significantly differ.

In summary, the above studies are inconclusive, with some of them attributing negative, and some, positive effects on children who have been labelled.
Other studies found no effect of labelling *per se* in the formation of attitudes
towards disabled individuals. The notion of positive effects, however, as it has
been presented in the majority of the above studies, is quite disturbing. How
'positive' can interactions be that include notions of pity, overprotectiveness,
dependency, 'special dispensation' and the perpetuation of 'sick roles'? The
response to this question has been offered by numerous disabled people, who
are the first to be affected by such 'positive' labelling effects and interactions
(Finkelstein 1980; Brisenden 1986; Oliver 1987; Harry 1991; Jones 1991;
Kefala 1991; Verity 1991; Morris 1992).

Additionally, the studies mentioned earlier have isolated the creation and
formation of labelling from the institutionalized practices of the society that
created such labels in the first place. As some of these studies were mainly
experimental, they did not pay attention to the reasons and the social roots
behind the creation of such labels. The question raised by Oliver (1992b)
regarding the consequences of integrating children into an education system
which reflects and reinforces inequality is highly important. The creation of
labelling has been associated with wider and complex ideological assumptions
and myths that are to be found within institutions such as schools:

> The problem is to adjust unsatisfactory pupils to satisfactory schools . . .
> Pupils are failing to adjust satisfactorily to schools is the verdict, and the
> necessary remedy is to modify this behaviour, to replace the unsatis-
> factory responses by more appropriate social behaviour (or at least place
> them in a room in which their influence on the rest of the school popu-
> lace will be minimal) using positive and negative stimuli devised by a
> skilled modifier.
>
> (Barton and Meighan 1979: 1)

In the book *Schools, Pupils and Deviance* (Barton and Meighan 1979), a
number of authors have shown how deviancy and labelling is a creation of
institutional climates – an issue that the majority of the earlier-mentioned
studies failed to take on board. Further, there are other studies that have
shown that 'Even if teachers set out to treat children as individuals, they are

constrained by circumstances to label them in terms of categories reflecting institutional necessities and external pressures' (Hargreaves *et al.* 1975; Sharp and Green 1975, cited in Quicke *et al.* 1990: 35).

Finally, in exploring the effect of labelling in peers' and teachers' attitudes and how labelling affects disabled childrens' lives, Karagiannis claims that

> Handicapped [*sic*] children have been stereotyped by 'non-handicapped' children as less capable, less assertive, unattractive academically and behaviourally problematic, unhappy, non-conforming, withdrawn, requiring supervision, and opposing peers. Labelling persons using the above characterizations has serious impact in their lives. On one hand they are forced to perceive themselves as useless in society. On the other hand, by socially devaluating them through social stigmata we reduce their chances to participate in the community and prove that they are not what their social stigmata have characterized them. Therefore, they are unwillingly involved in a vicious circle as a shifting of others' attitudes cannot be accomplished without interaction.
>
> (Karagiannis 1988: 89)

This view has been supported by Quicke *et al.* (1990: 35), who point out that deviant labelling 'contributes to the maintenance of a social climate where pupils are not treated with equal respect either by peers or by teachers – a climate, therefore, which is a breeding ground for prejudice'. In a microlevel analysis, labelling is associated with interpersonal behaviour in that the concepts of self and social roles are both learned in personal relationships. It has been argued that the self is 'penetrated' by others whom we meet and by their responses to us (Thomas 1978). For a disabled person the basic means by which the self is evaluated has been qualitatively different from the experience of the majority. For instance, Thomas (1978) has argued that interpersonal communication between disabled and non-disabled children has been greatly influenced by two types of 'deviance': primary and secondary deviance. Primary deviance, according to Thomas, is linked with the practical difficulties in interpersonal relationships deriving from the impairment itself, which are accompanied by social stigmatization and stereotyping, thus continuing secondary deviance.

The issue of social relationships between disabled and non-disabled children in integrated settings has been investigated by a number of studies from two points of view. One set of studies looked at the social adjustment of disabled children in integrated settings by measuring their self-concept and sociometric status, 'comparing' it with the self-concept and status of children in segregated settings. Another set of studies has focused on measuring or exploring peers' attitudes towards and interactions with disabled children. Both sets of studies have used social relationships as a criterion of 'assessing' the social benefits of the integration process; I shall now look at the main findings of these studies.

Social relationships between disabled and non-disabled children

In the initial phase of the integration process, the main tendency was to examine the process of integration from the perspective of disabled children's social adjustment within integrated settings. Social adjustment data are mainly of two kinds, self-concept and sociometric status. Investigators who have compared the self-concepts of students who attended special classes with students who attended ordinary classes have reported conflicting results, with some finding no significant differences and others reporting significant differences favouring either children who have been educated in segregated schools or children educated in ordinary schools.

Carroll (1967) and Mayrowitz (1962) found that students in partially segregated settings showed more improvement than students in segregated settings. A possible explanation for this finding is that children having a dual reference group of both disabled and non-disabled students are able to gain satisfaction from knowing that they, too, are as capable as a group of other children (i.e. their segregated classmates). Much earlier studies reflecting the dominant ideologies of their time have argued that children had better self-concepts when they were fully segregated (Cassidy and Stanton 1959; Thurston 1959).

Even though the above studies are not recent they serve the purpose of showing how futile and problematic was the debate in the research area regarding integration versus segregation processes. First, this type of work provides a whole series of operational, conceptual and analytical problems. The concept of 'social adjustment' and the development of self-concept/esteem were perceived as context-free processes with little recognition that in a very fundamental sense the self is a product of a person's interaction with others. Decontextualizing the formation of self-concept tended to belittle the importance of the social environment in which the meaning of such a concept had been developed in the first place. Second, another concern derives from the way complex issues such as the formation of self-concept/esteem were approached. It is questionable whether the nature of a person's experience, her interpretation of her surroundings, the meaning of her statements and the nature of her emotions can be quantified on a rating scale of self-esteem. Third, conclusions such as 'children had better self-concepts when they were fully segregated' tended to be self-justifying, scarcely recognizing that such conclusions were based on doubtful comparisons that have failed to offer an account of the social and cultural worlds of the persons under investigation. Thus on the one hand they tended to justify segregated practices and legitimize a deficit model of disabled people; on the other they contributed little to the struggle to use integration as a means to create a more inclusive understanding of the educational community.

Other empirical studies concentrated on the highly important issue of interactions and/or patterns of interactions between disabled children and their peers. Cavallaro and Porter (1980) studied children's choice of partner in free play. They found that friendship patterns of ordinary children were such that they tended to have one partner who they consistently chose, but disabled children did not seem to have such strong relationships. Guralnick and Croom (1980) also examined the degree of social interactions within a group of preschool students. In the group non-disabled, mildly, moderately, and severely 'handicapped' children were included. With adults constructing play situations it was found that (a) moderately and severely 'handicapped' children interacted with all four subgroups of children, (b) non-disabled and mildly 'handicapped' children interacted more frequently among each other than was expected by the researchers; and (c) non-disabled and mildly 'handicapped' children interacted less frequently with moderately and severely 'handicapped' children than expected.

Another study investigating the inclinations of non-disabled children to help their disabled peers found that overall the 'orthopedically handicapped children' were selected first, more often than children with Down's Syndrome (Kennedy *et al.* 1982). The reasons given by the young participants for their choices varied. This study found that the notion that a disabled individual should be helped seems to occur quite early (i.e. at around 8 years old), while children have an inclination to offer more help to a disabled child who appears to be the 'most needy'. In addition it was found that children ascribed negative status to disabled children by referring to them as 'babies', 'young' and 'small'. In a more recent study where social integration was measured by the frequency with which disabled children interacted with their peers, it was found that there were fewer interactions than could be expected by chance alone (Jenkins *et al.* 1989).

The above findings were similar to earlier studies examining peers' acceptance scores among each other and between them and disabled students. They found that the scores of acceptance were significantly lower when referring to disabled children than non-disabled peers. Additionally, it was found that the degree of isolation of disabled children steadily increased the lower down the intellectual scale one went (Baldwin 1958; Jordan 1959).

These findings can be interpreted in another way as well. They indicate that the nature of social isolation that disabled children had experienced at the initial phase of integrational practices (in the 1960s) was not qualitatively altered in the 1980s, despite the rhetoric surrounding integrational policies and practices.

However, it will be misleading to assume that integration is static and has not brought any attitudinal changes. There are studies that have investigated the influence of disabled and non-disabled children's interactions on the attitudes and understanding of non-disabled towards disabled people. These studies have indicated that contact with disabled children influences non-disabled children's attitudes. Specifically, Sheare (1974) found in an experimental study that the group of children who were assigned to non-academic classes with disabled children revealed more positive attitude ratings on the acceptance scale than the control group of children who had not been integrated in classes with disabled children. Further, McHale and Simeonsson (1980) showed that contact with 'severely handicapped' students improved non-disabled students' 'understanding' of their disabled peers.

Rynders *et al.* (1980) showed that the way the activities are structured influences the nature of interactions among disabled and non-disabled children. According to that study, the cooperative structure promoted significantly more positive and inclusive interactions and attitudes. That cooperative learning experiences promote positive interactions and friendships between non-disabled and disabled peers has been reported in another study by Johnson and Johnson (1981). The cooperative structuring of learning activities, when accompanied by information/knowledge to peers about disability issues, provides a background for the creation of positive attitudes of young children towards their disabled peers (Lewis and Lewis 1988). Knowledge and awareness regarding disability issues have been characterized as key features in changing negative peer attitudes towards disabled children (Shapiro and Morgolis 1988). In addition, Lynas (1986) pointed out that teachers should be careful about the amount of help they offer to disabled children and the way this help is offered to them. Positive discrimination, if not presented carefully, can have socially segregating effects by reinforcing negative peer attitudes.

However, attitudes seem to be a much more complicated affair. This was shown by a study which endeavoured to examine the attitudes of secondary school pupils towards the notion of mental retardation. The results indicated a confusion about the nature and causes of 'mental retardation'. It also indicated that the same person held conflicting feelings and opinions regarding integration and interactions with disabled people (Kyle and Davies 1991). Other studies have demonstrated that attitudes towards and interactions of non-disabled with disabled people are affected by other parameters such as age, gender, class, race, and level of perceived competence that the non-disabled child holds. Gender was especially highlighted as a social parameter influencing the nature of attitudes (Goodman *et al.* 1972; Thomas 1978; Sandberg 1982; Firth and Rapley 1990).

Specifically, it has been emphasized by Quicke (1989; Quicke *et al.* 1990) that attitudinal research should take into consideration the impact of gender when children are asked to reveal their opinions and feelings regarding interactions with disabled children:

A number of quantitative attitudinal studies have suggested that in relation to all forms of handicap females demonstrate more 'positive' attitudes than males . . . Explanations for these findings have been various, but usually refer either to psycho-biological 'within child' factors or to role socialized traits . . . Such findings would suggest that cultural studies might help to illuminate attitudes to mental handicap by examining the relationship between integration policies and the establishment of gender identities.

(Quicke *et al.* 1990: 32–3)

The above studies are only a small sample of the type of investigations that have been conducted in the areas of social integration and peers' attitudes towards interactions with disabled children. The majority of studies focused on the degree rather than the nature, the meaning(s) and the quality of interactions between disabled and non-disabled children. Peer rejection was a fairly common pattern according to the evidence of these studies, indicating that peers' attitudes were influenced by a number of variables. Disabled children's 'ability' or 'inability' to form relationships, peers' perceptions of a disabled person, peers' perceptions of a disabled child's academic performance, the amount of actual interaction with disabled children, the type of learning activities within which both disabled and non-disabled children interact, and the age, gender and class of the peers have been identified by previous attitudinal research as being some of the variables influencing peers' attitudes towards their disabled classmates. However, the majority of these studies have isolated each of these variables from their social and cultural contexts and in so doing they have belittled their complexity. Complex relationships have been summarized in conclusive statements, often with little or no explanation of the 'why's' and 'how's' necessary for understanding the creation and meaning of different social patterns. At times the dominant language used in the majority of these studies was in itself offensive and disablist while concepts such as 'social interactions' and 'social acceptability' were often ill-defined, generating a dependency deficit model with regard to disabled children.

The majority of the above studies used the 'assessment' of the social acceptability of disabled children as one of several criteria to evaluate the effectiveness of the integration process. Another set of studies has focused on teachers' attitudes towards integration in evaluating the integration process. These studies are based on a recognition that positive teacher attitudes are the most important factors in ensuring the success of integration; I shall now turn to the main findings of these investigations.

Teachers' attitudes towards the integration process

There are a number of studies which have examined integration from the teachers' perspective. The findings on this issue are inconclusive with some studies (mainly conducted in United States) reporting negative teachers' attitudes towards integrating disabled students (Baker and Gottlieb 1980; Leyser and Abrams 1983; Feldman and Altman 1985) and some others reporting positive attitudes (Hegarty and Pocklington 1981; Pinhas and Schmelkin 1989). Thomas (1985) identified numerous factors, both institutional and personal, which in combination may serve as predictors of teachers' attitudes towards integrating disabled children. Some of these factors were: the traditional school policy regarding integration, policy of allocation of students to classes (mixed ability or streaming), the head teacher's attitude to integration, the quality of support offered by the contact special educator, the relationship between the mainstream and the support teacher (their roles and their ascribed responsibilities), conservatism as a dimension of the teacher's personality, gender, type of teaching, and teacher's level of confidence in selecting appropriate teaching methods for disabled children.

Another study (Bowman 1989) aimed to review teacher-training in the context of a variety of country systems (in 14 countries); to consider teachers' attitudes to integration; and to produce a report which could form the basis of meetings about teacher training and integration. The results were significantly relevant to integration. In each of the five UNESCO world regions it was found that teachers' perceptions of integration differed significantly across and within countries according to various factors: the existence or not of a mandate law favouring integration, the amount and type of their training, their experience of pupils with potentially 'handicapping' conditions, and the support available in ordinary schools. Specifically, it was found that teachers' attitudes were positive towards the integration of 'delicate' students (75.5 per cent), physical 'handicap' students (63 per cent), students with specific learning difficulties (54 per cent), students with speech 'defect' (50 per cent); while they revealed less positive attitudes towards the integration of students with severe mental handicap (*sic*) (2.5 per cent) and students with multiple handicaps (*sic*) (7.5 per cent). This study was based on a 'hierarchy of preference' list of disability groups which has also been used in other studies (for example, Hegarty and Pocklington 1981). There are two crucial issues revealed by these two studies. First, teachers do categorize children according to their specific impairment; second, mentally disabled children are at the bottom of the teachers' preference list. Moreover, the findings of this study revealed that teachers' attitudes are influenced by the forms of help and support that they receive. The link between the formation of attitudes and the nature and the quality of support that teachers receive in their working environment has been substantiated by other studies (Thomas 1985; Karagiannis 1988).

Finally, there are a number of other characteristics that have been identified as influential on the formation of teachers' attitudes towards integration. These are related more to personal/demographic characteristics of teachers, such as age and amount of teaching experience with disabled people. Specifically, it has been reported that younger educators and educators with a greater amount of teaching experience with disabled children tended to have more positive attitudes towards integration (Stainback *et al.* 1984). It seems, however, that these characteristics are not so strong in influencing attitudes. Reynolds *et al.* (1982) did not find any significant differences in teachers' responses towards integration when compared on the basis of teacher ages, teaching experiences, and teaching experiences with disabled children.

All these empirical findings provide us with a mass of information that we should be aware of when involved in attitudinal studies regarding integration. However, as already mentioned (see Introduction), attitudinal research in the area of special needs raises serious questions, such as how do we define attitudes? and most important of all, how do we proceed in exploring them? The response to such questions involves theoretical/ideological problems, tensions and tangles of thought in a complex interface between various theories about attitudes *per se,* and integration, as well as lived experience in the field. The following analysis, originating mainly from an American positivist epistemological position explores the fundamental theoretical principles underlying the examination (and measuring) of attitudes from a conventional 'objective' perspective. Familiarity with the ideological/methodological logic under-pinning the dominant patterns of attitudinal research is necessary before proceeding to a broader critical perspective. Thus the discussion will initially focus on the literature related to the general theoretical/methodological basis for the term 'attitude'.

An examination of the term 'attitude'

A variety of meanings have been given to the term 'attitude' during its history. Initially, the term 'attitude' was used as a jargon term for artists to describe body position in painting. Later, though, that term was used by Darwin to describe a stereotypic behavioural motoric response associated with the expression of an emotion (in Kahle 1984). In 1906 Charles Sherrington referred to attitudes as a continuous state, and not as an occasional outburst as was defined by Darwin. Therefore, according to Sherrington, 'attitude reflected the stable nature of body position' (in Kahle 1984: 3). In the German language a similar term was developed, *aufgabe,* that was usually translated as mind-set rather than attitude. Margaret Wasburn attempted to integrate Sherrington's concept of attitude with the concept of *aufgabe* by proposing a theory of incipient action, of learning by doing. As Kahle stated, this development helped to establish one element of the eventual term 'attitude'. Golstein, by criticizing Sherrington's thinking, provided a second element of the term 'attitude'. According to Golstein, imagination, creative thinking and the ability of humans to be concerned with the possibilities of life should be part of this term. William Thomas expounded upon the meaning of the term, defining attitudes as 'a process of individual consciousness in the social world' (in Kahle 1984: 3). As Kahle claimed, 'Thomas formulated a vision of the attitude concept that more or less persists until today, he perhaps unwittingly removed the psychological element and, therefore, the observable element of an attitude.'

Other authors (Thurston 1928; Likert 1932), in operationalizing the term 'attitude' for research purposes, claimed that attitudes are nothing more or nothing less than what the attitude scale measures. Operationally, attitudes were mainly defined as a matter of preference.

This battle over defining 'attitudes' continued to be of great importance. Actually one of the major epistemological positions within the traditional positivist way of thinking was to operationalize their concepts and to define them in terms of either measurable behaviour or in terms of measurable variables. The conceptual or operational definition of the term 'attitudes' has been one of the major problems in social psychology for more than half a century. Possible explanations of such a difficulty have been offered; one such reason is that attitudes are constructs rather than concepts. As Cameron and Whetten stated,

> Constructs are abstractions that exist in the heads of people but they have no object reality. They cannot be pin-pointed, counted or observed. They exist only because they are inferred from the results of observable phenomena. They are mental abstractions designed to give meaning to ideas or interpretations. One difference between constructs and concepts is that concepts can be defined and exactly specified by observing objective events. Constructs cannot be so specified.
>
> (Cameron and Whetten 1983: 7)

Other authors have suggested that attitudes are difficult to define because of their multidimensional character, which includes a variety of cognitive, affective and conative components (Fishbein and Ajzen 1974). The operational formulation of the term included three elements as components: the affective or evaluative dimension (good–bad), activity dimension (active–passive), and the potency or cognitive dimension (strong–weak).

Later in the historical development definitions became more abstract and ambiguous, while attitude was perceived as some 'inaccessible entity in the "black box" of the individual' (Roiser 1974: 112) that can be measured somehow with complicated behaviouristic measures. Characteristically, it was claimed that

> A person's attitude toward an object can be estimated by multiplying his evaluation of each attribute associated with the object by his subjective probability that the object has that attribute, and then summing the products for the total set of beliefs. Similarly, a person's attitude toward a behaviour can be estimated by multiplying his evaluation of each of the behaviour's consequences by his subjective probability that performing that behaviour will lead to that consequence, and then summing the products for the total set of belief.
>
> (Fishbein and Ajzen 1975: 223)

There were other theorists who, even though they perceived attitudes as abstractions, linked them directly with the environment:

> Attitudes are adaptation abstractions, or generalizations, about functioning in the environment, especially the social environment, that are expressed as predispositions to evaluate an object, concept or symbol. This abstraction process emerges continuously from the assimilation, accommodation, and organization of environmental information, by individuals in order to promote interchanges between the individual and the environment that from the individual's perspective, are favourable to preservation and optimal functioning.
>
> (Kahle 1984: 5)

Even though attitudes were linked with a social environment they were rather perceived from an individualistic perspective. The emphasis was on accommodating or assimilating information into already existent mental structures. The key feature was not conflict but generalization, which promoted adaptability for a better functioning into different environments.

According to the conventional attitudinal logic, in order to be objective, researchers must bear in mind that when examining these generalizations they are restricted to analyse attitudes in relation to the specific action, the target, at which the action is directed, the context in which the action is performed, and the time at which it is performed (Ajzen and Fishbein 1977). Thus, a specific action must be insulated and separated from the wider environment – with no involvement of relationships and interactions – if attitudes are to be measured.

Another issue has arisen from positivistic logic regarding attitudinal research, which has actually become one of the fundamental problems in social psychology, namely the question of attitude–behaviour consistency. This concern was based on the assumption that if there is no relationship between expressed attitudes and behaviour then there is no point attempting to understand attitudes (see Bentler and Speckart 1981). There has been an ongoing debate about the value of measuring attitudes, as predictors of overt behaviour, if there are low or non-significant relations between attitudinal predictors and behavioural criteria.

However, social psychology has witnessed a revival of interest in the relationship between attitudes and action (Ajzen and Fishbein 1977). Some authors have responded to the accumulated evidence of attitude–behaviour inconsistency by suggesting conceptual and methodological refinements intended to increase the likelihood of correspondence between attitude and action. They were engaged with the issue of the causal effect of attitudes on behaviours versus that of behaviours on attitudes. It has been reported that

> Investigators have taken four different positions concerning causal relationships between attitudes and behaviours: attitudes cause behaviours (McGuire, 1976); behaviours cause attitudes (Bem, 1972); attitudes and behaviours have mutual causal impact (Kelman, 1974) and attitudes and behaviours are slightly if at all, related.
>
> (in Bentler and Speckart 1981: 226)

Other authors reached a consensus according to which attitudes should be conceptualized as underlying dispositions which determine, along with other influences, a variety of behaviours toward an object (Tognacci *et al.* 1974). So attitude was considered to be only one of many factors determining behaviour. This work represented a shift in the focus of research efforts, a shift from examining whether or not attitudes are related to behaviour to examining the conditions under which attitudes and behaviour co-vary (Weigel and Newman 1976).

Fishbein and Ajzen (1974) and Ajzen and Fishbein (1977) made an attempt to integrate discrepant findings in their thorough exploration of the research literature on the attitude–behaviour relationship. They found that people's actions are systematically related to their attitudes only when the nature of the attitude predictors and behavioural criteria are taken into consideration. After defining the four elements that constitute attitudinal and behavioural entities – action, target at which the action is directed, the context in which the action is performed, and the time at which it is performed – they suggested that 'The strength of an attitude–behaviour relationship depends in large part on the degree of correspondence between attitudinal and behavioural entities' (Ajzen and Fishbein 1977: 891).

In the positivistic logic tradition of measuring attitudes Ajzen and Fishbein (1977) suggested that a researcher would have to take a closer look at the behavioural criteria. They suggested three behavioural terms: a single-act criterion for a behaviour delineated according to a specific action, target, time and place; a repeated observation criterion generalized across different targets, times or places; and a multi-act criterion further generalized across different actions. Although a global attitudinal predisposition may not be related to any particular single-act criterion, it will be significantly related to a repeated-observation or multiple-act criterion if target, action and context are at identical levels of specificity in attitudinal and behavioural measures (in Bentler and Speckart 1979). Thus experimental and control environments were required in order to obtain identical levels of specificity in attitudinal and behavioural measures. Such a methodological logic demanded the control of the environment, by requesting participants to take a specific role, respond to certain questions and further respond in certain ways predetermined by the researcher. In turn this logic created the assumption that researchers ought to be 'neutral', 'objective' and 'ideologically detached' from the topic they had identified for examination, so as not to 'jeopardize' the objectivity of the study. However, my experiences during the course of the research – and the ideological/theoretical tensions involved – largely did not reflect these principles. This realization was strengthened after reading accounts which included an alternative, rather than conventional, methodological stance (Hargreaves 1972; Berger and Mohr 1976; Cohen and Taylor 1976; Davies 1982; Dunn 1991; Pollard 1992). These were accounts in which the aims and the arguments were not only valid and strong but also offered a deeper understanding of everyday complex social relationships. At the same time, my contact with accounts written by disabled people challenged my own pre-assumptions about issues of disability and led me to question the assumptions involved in the way attitudes towards disabled people have been examined with attitudinal research.

A critical reflection on conventional attitudinal research

Quantitative empirical research mainly conducted in American contexts using conventional attitudinal measures seems to have examined most of the areas of integration (i.e. effectiveness of integration versus segregation, peers' interactions with disabled children, teachers' and peers' attitudes towards integration) in a quite mechanical way. Even though this type of research showed that results are inconclusive and that some groups of children seemed to evoke more negative attitudes in their teachers and/or their peers than others, they did not shed light on the context in which such attitudes were developed in the first place.

Further, like Mehan,

> I felt that large scale surveys and experiments masked important theoretical and policy issues, were ill-equipped to uncover the root causes of inequality and did not enable us to hear the voices of the disenfranchised. I thought that it was necessary to look much more closely at social life and listen to the voices of the dispossessed to understand the complex processes composing inequality.
>
> (Mehan 1993: 94)

Going back to the methodological procedures of some of the above attitudinal research conducted with the aid of conventional attitudinal measures I realized that attitudes were perceived as quantifiable stimuli and that they could be measured on precise scales with a 'high degree of objectivity' and generalizability. Integration was perceived as an unproblematic notion usually specified by the researchers. Comparisons were made between children educated in segregated settings with children educated in integrated settings, as if the two settings and the children's experiences were comparable.

Unnatural control and experimental settings were considered to be sufficient for measuring value-judgements. Justifying the above logic, Siperstein *et al.* (1988: 24) stated that 'a step-wise multiple regression analysis showed that children's attitudes towards the target child in the laboratory setting were related to their sociometric choices of the retarded classmate'.

Within the same conventional logic, labelling and competence were seen as independent variables that had, or did not have, an influence on the dependent variable attitudes. This mechanical behaviouristic treatment of attitudes was far from my understanding of attitudes as being a complex phenomenon, often inconsistent, influenced by different social parameters with unpredictable outcomes.

I do not mean to argue that research using conventional positivistic methods is of no value in our understanding of social phenomena. My dissatisfaction rather stemmed from the unproblematic way that both the terms 'attitudes' and 'integration' were used. It also stemmed from an emerging belief that our methodological tools construct the topic itself. Further, the nature of the topic influences and is influenced by the type of methods we use.

A further dissatisfaction with a lot of the articles of empirical research that I read originated from the aims of the research. If its aim, as claimed, was to enable teachers and peers to understand the processes in which they operate and to make sense of their experience then I could hardly see what could be the contribution of such structured experimental research. Experiences, meanings and definition of situations as well as formulation of ideas and restructuring of these ideas are much more complex than they were presented in quantifiable research. As Armistead (1974: 15) stated, 'With the best of scientific intentions, it [psychological social psychology] has left itself high and dry by ignoring social contexts which should not be taken for granted'.

In summary, attitude has been perceived as an entity that has to be detached from its relationships with other social entities in order to be measured. Sometimes this entity has been perceived as inaccessible because it resides somewhere in the individual (the subconscious); it also includes a biological and a habitual dimension. There are, however, some general principles that can be described and applied to any situation as long as we can quantify and standardize them with highly sophisticated measurements. According to conventional attitude measures this can happen when we have operationalized the dependent variable attitude; the statements 'emanating' from it can be seen as simple stimuli from which the larger attitude is inferred. (For an extensive analysis, see Roiser's (1974) article, 'Asking silly questions'.) The next step is to find, whenever this is possible, a kind of a causal or deterministic relationship between verbal responses and overt actions, treating and perceiving this relationship as having a mechanical stimulus–response connection. For this to proceed, an attitude item should be precise, unambiguous and concrete otherwise it cannot be valid. If the relationship is not strong and significant then attitudinal dichotomous responses are of low value.

Thus attitudes have been abstracted from the context in which they were developed in the first place, and so they become apolitical, asocial and ahistorical. Any involvement of ideologies and social, cultural, or moral parameters may jeopardize the objectivity of the study – the researcher can be accused of not being value-free. The role of the researcher here is crucial, as according to the conventional positivistic logic s/he has to be a *tabula rasa*, excluding her/his subjectivity and any other leading interpretation. S/he has to be 'neutral' and 'detached' from the events.

This rationale seems to be limited and limiting because it fails to take into consideration that social phenomena are not events in the outside world perceived by passive observers, but interpretations by an active subject who defines the field, who affects and is affected by the environment in which s/he participates, acting intentionally in relation to that environment (see Armistead 1974). Conventional positivist logic also fails to recognize that the nature of the vexed topic of attitudes and integration is highly political, cultural, historical and social.

Attitude is a social entity that encompasses ways of thinking, ways of feeling and experiences that are developed in specific interdependent cultural contexts. Thus measuring attitudes means measuring people's thoughts, opinions and experiences. The notion of experience here is not the same as the notion of overt behaviour that researchers strive to measure and afterwards connect with verbally expressed opinions to figure out if there is any consistency. Experience is a broader term which includes behaviour in relation to the way the participant feels about it, understands it, interprets it and even evaluates it. The first problematic issue derives from the question that Armistead stated: 'Does a lifetime's stigmatization reflect itself in where a black person marks a rating scale of self esteem? . . . Can you quantify the nature of a person's experience, his interpretation of his surroundings, the meaning of his statements, the nature of his emotions?' (Armistead 1974: 19). Decontextualized, polarized dichotomous responses of agreement and/or disagreement about complex phenomena become alienated knowledge to the researcher – but most of all to the participants and their lives.

On the one hand, it becomes alienated knowledge for the researcher because, as Armistead pointed out,

> If you spend your time concentrating upon variations aren't you likely to forget about the nature of what you are studying and why it is there in the first place? For instance, if you set about accounting for variations in prejudice won't you tend to ignore the nature and meaning of prejudice as a social phenomenon and what this might tell us about why there is prejudice at all?
>
> (Armistead 1974: 19)

On the other hand it becomes alienated knowledge to the participants because of their passive position towards a stage of a research process that is detached from all the other research stages.

There are other consequences for both the researcher and the researched. From the researcher's point of view s/he thinks that the predefined statements offered to the participants do not include any moral assumptions and that they have been checked so as to be clear and non-biased. However, this is not the case. A statement 'Every "handicapped" person should be treated equally in an educational setting' reflects the attitude of the researcher. There are going to be participants (especially disabled participants) who would claim that such a statement uses a disabling language. Additionally it is ambiguous because equality is a complex contingent phenomenon subject to different interpretations.

From the participant's point of view, s/he is caught in a prespecified context with little or no space to voice her/his objections or comment upon the statement. Both the expression of attitudes and the concrete actions are subject to a range of contingencies. 'As any interviewer will tell you, people just do not want to answer specific-sounding questions in general terms; their attitude is enshrined in the interviewer's bugbear "it all depends"' (Heritage 1974: 98). Thus attitude scales typically comprise of a number of brief predefined statements that tend to be fraught with value-judgements, that ignore the meaning of the situation to the participants, depoliticize the social context and treat participants as passive respondents abstracted from any ongoing real-life contexts and processes.

In the case in which the researcher measures behaviour, what happens when the same behaviour has different meanings for different actors displaying the behaviour? Further, what happens when the interpretation the researcher offers for an overt behaviour is far from the interpretation ascribed to the behaviour by either the person who exhibited it or by the persons who are affected by it?

Thus a fundamental principle underlying the methodological and analytical/interpretative procedures of this study is the recognition that attitude is a complex social phenomenon which includes ideologies, thoughts, feelings and experiences. It can be seen as

> A communicative act, aimed at defining the relationship between people or groups . . . The attitude and its statements are all part of a debate . . . The debates between attitudinal groups are grounded in the real problems of the social world. The resolution is thus an extremely slow process, depending on the ability of particular groups to succeed in overcoming the problems they set themselves.
>
> (Armistead 1974: 112)

Overt behaviour is not an automatic response to a stimulus based on the existence of a non-accessible 'black box'. It is, rather, connected with the ideology that a person holds and brings into the working environment in relation to the structural constraints that an institutionalized environment imposes upon that person.

Social relationships and interactions in everyday life are key features because they affect, shape or even structure identities, and vice versa. Exploring relationships at a microlevel helps us to understand, or at least to try to understand, how we make sense of the events that affect our lives; it can even help us to identify what has been internalized and taken for granted as 'natural'.

In every social interaction we exhibit attitudes, in how we define the interaction (the situation), what we believe, and what we feel about it – including the ways we choose to behave towards something or someone. As Armistead (1974: 20) notes, 'The social is not just something that occurs when people meet, but is involved more deeply in our very thoughts and identities.'

In more complex situations what we believe and what we feel is in contrast to how we act. In these cases our actions are not 'authentic'. There are tensions created in the relationship between the self and the surrounding superordinate reality. A better explanation and understanding of the reasons behind this inconsistency can be offered by an examination of the institutional constraints (structural, situational, personal, ideological) that the environment imposes on the person. How does the individual make sense of this environment and the social relationships involved?

Thus the micro-interactional analysis of everyday life can be complemented by a macro-analysis as both levels dialectically interact. It is important to mention here that, as Fulcher (1989a) has powerfully shown, policies are being made at different levels. Therefore it was necessary to avoid thinking of attitudes as a consensus among groups. I wanted to understand how different participants in the study made sense of what they were experiencing, what was the reason and justification behind their interaction, what were their definitions, myths, prejudices, opinions and feelings. I was strongly influenced in this decision by an analysis of attitudes from Roiser (1974) and Quicke *et al.* (1990). The first author showed how conventional measures exclude alternative ways of thinking by trying to achieve a consensus measure taking the line of least resistance among the groups battling to define the situation. He also referred to studies on deviancy in sociology, which even though they have received a fair amount of criticism, at least show that there are people who do not (or do not *want* to) subscribe to the dominant or popular consensus, regardless of the consequences. The second authors stressed the point that we are unable to understand and, more importantly, evaluate attitudes if we are not aware of the reasons behind their existence.

However, there was one more strong assumption that shaped the design of this study – disability is a product of social interactions between people with impairments and the way others respond to them. That is, there are long-standing and powerful social continuities, traditions and relationships that define a person with an impairment as a disabled person. Disabled persons' identities have already been defined 'for them by us' in the most discriminatory and derogatory way.

As researchers we may share the responsibility of perpetuating discrimination towards disabled people by the very nature of our questions and the methods we use. Because of our attitudes, on the one hand we claim that research into attitudes regarding disability has as an ultimate aim the exploration of others' attitudes so as to contribute to policy-making and help make a more positive and inclusive environment. On the other hand we tend to ignore what disabled people so strongly advocate. And what they advocate is that if researchers do not take into consideration disabled people's voices then the research is much more harmful and discriminatory.

There are a lot of accounts written by disabled people which can enable non-disabled researchers to proceed in non-discriminatory research. In his article 'Re-defining disability: a challenge to research', Oliver (1987) stated that research on disability has too often failed to involve disabled people except, for example, as passive subjects of interviews and observations drawn up by non-disabled researchers and based upon able-bodied assumptions. He pointed out that much research on disability has contributed little or nothing to improving the quality of life of disabled people as well as to influencing social policies.

Finkelstein (1980) stated that even where researchers have focused upon social factors like attitudes of the able-bodied or stigma, they have still seen these factors as being causally related to the impaired individual. Further, Trieschmann (1980) claims that disabled people have felt victimized by professionals who write articles about reactions to disability that are based more upon theory than fact. However, even the notion of facts has been problematized by other disabled people when they lead to a partial and inhibiting view of the disabled individual. Brisenden has extensively analysed the demand to look beyond fragmented facts, especially the medical 'facts':

Presumably it is possible, under certain conditions, to isolate a set of 'facts', in the form of a list of general physical or intellectual character-istics, that apply to each form of disability. But the use of these is limited as there cannot be a formula derived from them that will cope with the particular needs of each individual. Indeed, taken alone, the 'facts' may lead only to distortion and misunderstanding and to a view of disabled people as a category of rejects, as people flawed in some aspect of their humanity.

(Brisenden 1986: 1)

Within this context of creating studies and formulating facts, the researcher is neither detached nor objective, neither neutral nor natural. S/he enters the field with fears, anxieties, uncertainties, problems of ethical integrity (see Appendix 1) and presumptions which are evolving or even changing throughout the process. His/her stance and the complexities of the context – as well as the structural constraints – influence the decision-making and the nature of the research (Vlachou 1995a). This study has been strongly influ-enced by the insight that the selection of different methods is related to the way we define aspects of the 'paramount reality' (see Cohen and Taylor 1976) within which both the researcher and the participants act. As Schratz (1993: 57) has indicated, 'It is not so much the scientific design that determines the research findings but the interactions among the people involved.'

In the book so far I have considered some theoretical aspects regarding issues of disability, integration and attitudinal research production. This com-pletes the first analytical part of the book, which has built on critiques devel-oped over the past 15 years to explore the effects of policies, practices and ideologies which perpetuate exclusive structures. Now it is necessary to understand the structures within which weaker social groups continue to experience discrimination and exclusion; I want to explore the relationships between microlevels of action in schools and classrooms and macrostruc-tures/mechanisms by which the term 'special' is socially constructed.

The study now considers the case of one primary school that had a policy of integrating, in a cross-sectional way, 40 pupils identified as having special educational needs, including six children with Down's Syndrome. Taking the perspective that the individual, her/his sense of identity and her/his behav-iour are produced and shaped through social interactions, I was searching for a methodological design that would enable me to make sense of these pro-cesses in a 'natural' social environment. That is, I had to 'merge' myself in this environment and communicate formally and informally with partici-pants, allowing space for participants to express their own understanding about integration and interactions with disabled children (for an extended analysis see Vlachou 1995a). As a result, the research involved extensive par-ticipant observation for more than one-and-a-half years, semistructured interviews and informal discussions with 19 teachers, as well as individual and group discussions (with the use of a photograph) with 103 pupils (see Appendices 2 and 3).

Parts 2 and 3 focus on the reality of everyday life within an educational setting, in which a collection of people try to make sense of this reality, their relationships, and the tensions between themselves and their everyday educational life.

PART 2

TEACHERS' PERSPECTIVES

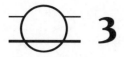 3

Teachers and the changing culture of teaching

Before focusing on an analysis of teachers' attitudes toward the process of integration, this chapter will begin by exploring the way teachers participating in the study experienced their job, and their feelings about the broader educational scene. This discussion is important for two main reasons. First, 'any critique of teaching or teachers must endeavour to understand the working conditions and constraints with which teachers are attempting to cope' (Barton 1987: 247; see also Barton and Walker 1981). Calls for teachers to promote more inclusive educational practices cannot be effectively met while teachers themselves experience conflicting constraints and expectations, insecurity and a general lack of encouragement. Second, almost every reference to integration in the interviews was linked inseparably with the wider educational context.

Of course, issues concerning teachers and teaching have a very long history in the sociology of education, probably because they are the most visible face of schooling. Teachers have been at the centre of a plethora of analyses and their profession has been viewed from many different perspectives. It has been argued that the general standing of teaching as an occupation, in contemporary societies, suffers from low or uncertain status. This has often been associated with a lack of specific and explicit technical modes of operating within the profession of teaching, together with the complexities involved in locating teachers within a social class structure (Lortie 1975; Ginsburg *et al.* 1980; Hunt 1990).

However, a key feature that differentiates teachers from other workers is that teaching, characteristically, involves various degrees of personal involvement, ideological commitment and investment of self (see Lortie 1975; Woods 1981, 1983; Woods and Pollard 1988; Pollard 1992). Additionally, as Jennifer Nias (1989) has argued, primary teaching is a complex and skilled activity, calling for a highly developed ability to hold in balance a multitude of demands and tensions. She argues that to 'feel like a teacher' is to learn to live with dilemma, contradiction and paradox and – at its best – to experience in their resolution the creative satisfactions of the artist. Because of these characteristics of their vocation, it is expected that teachers might have a well-developed sense of the way the constraints within which they have to work might affect them as human beings and as professionals.

Pollard's (1985, 1992) use of the notion of interests-at-hand provides a starting point for identifying, analysing and contextualizing some of the factors that influence teachers' perceptions and feelings about their job. He adopted Schutz's (1970, in Pollard 1992) concept of interests-at-hand to analyse from a symbolic interactionist point of view the element of self as it affects and is affected by everyday educational interactions. In his analysis of the social world of primary school, focusing particularly on enjoyment, workload, health and stress, and autonomy, he found that the most salient point was teachers' desire to control their work situation, particularly its effects on them personally. He concluded that these concerns were related to the maintenance of self-image.

His analysis in regard to the notion of interests-at-hand is important for understanding 'how priorities are perceived as classroom processes evolve' (Woods 1981: 283). These interests-at-hand will be incorporated into this discussion, but they will be considered in relation to the way that, in the study, they were being affected by current political and educational directives. The following transcribed material was derived from asking each teacher to talk about the way s/he experienced teaching, about what s/he liked or disliked. I will focus first on sources of satisfaction and enjoyment. Before doing so, however, it must be noted that most of the following responses originated from mainstream and not support teachers or child care assistants. This is probably because mainstream teachers' interests-at-hand were affected to a greater extent by the new political directives; mainstream teachers were in the forefront of implementing them and had to deal with a wider range of responsiblities. Support teachers were affected, too, by the new circumstances – but to a lesser degree and in a different way that will be explored later.

Satisfaction

It seemed that being in contact with children, with all its difficulties, had become 'a way of life' and had formed an important part of the identity of these primary school teachers:

> I like working with the children. I like the classroom environment. I would not like being an administrator because I like working with them [children], seeing them develop. I enjoy their company. It has become a way of life.

This was not unexpected as teachers' conception of their role cannot exist without the complementary role of pupils. Teachers' definitions of teaching included, primarily, being with children, building relationships with them, pursuing personal interests and contributing to the creation and/or development of identities. This last element was mentioned by the majority of teachers:

> I like to watch children blossom. I think it's lovely to take someone who cannot write, cannot read, or is perhaps struggling at that stage and gradually see them progress and really blossom. I like the way the world is open to them. They still have a sense of wonder around . . . I think it's wonderful to contribute to the process.

Contributing to the development of identities offers power, pride, satisfaction and responsibilities to the contributor who proves him/herself useful and his/her presence as being indispensable. The internal pleasure stems from the assumption that the teacher is one more member of the group called 'significant others' in children's lives. Of course teachers' perception of children and the way they think about children's performance is highly significant. It can be claimed that teachers view children as 'incomplete entities', which automatically offers them (teachers) power and authority over defining situations and proceeding in practices based on these conceptions:

> A lot of them would do nothing if left to it. They'll try to do as little and get away with it, you know, but if they'll be pushed they'll do it and they'll get something out of it at the end.

Power and authority is attributed to teachers (in relation to students) because all teachers have two basic sub-roles which they cannot escape: the roles of instructor and disciplinarian. The essential point here is that teachers obtained satisfaction (intellectual and personal) out of the enactment of these roles, which offered them the opportunity to be in contact with children and to contribute to their development.

The personal fulfilment and satisfaction derived from these roles has also been found in Nias's (1989) study in which 45 out of the 50 teachers involved saw themselves primarily as 'teachers' and went on to describe the way in which they were able to 'be themselves', 'be whole and be natural' through the enactment of their role. Nias (p. 89) further stated that 'my interviewees expressed very high levels of satisfaction with teaching as an occupation. Most when invited to name things they did not enjoy doing found it hard to go beyond mundane chores.' However, as Pollard (1992: 108) stated, 'these data [in Nias's study] were collected before the recent legislation and there are good grounds for believing that the pattern might not be repeated today – as the Education Reform Act of 1988 starts to take effect'.

Indeed, my interviewees found it very difficult to identify any other source of satisfaction. When asked to reflect on teaching as an occupation, the overwhelming majority started talking about the things they did not enjoy or found difficult to cope with. The overriding impression was of personal dissatisfaction, anger and frustration about the conditions within which they had to work.

Sources of dissatisfaction

Teachers' first interest-at-hand, *satisfaction*, seemed to be severely under-mined. The part of the job teachers found attractive and satisfying (that of being in contact with children) was adversely affected and became extremely difficult to accomplish because of the transformation in the educational context, which demanded a redefinition of their roles. The increasing significance of bureaucratic, commercial and economic priorities in the social activity of teaching assigned to teachers the role of paid bureaucratic servants who were expected to 'deliver the goods'. But teachers had a great difficulty in seeing themselves as bureaucrats – the role conflicted with their self-perception and actions, and brought a lot of tension and dissatisfaction:

> I was not trained to be a clerk – I was trained to teach children. I never intended to fill in papers. I never did secretarial work. Now you have to write everything down. There is so much paperwork that it detracts from the job you are supposed to do.

> It has become more difficult over the years with the things you are expected to do which aren't really concerned with teaching in the classroom.

> Teaching to me is about working with the kids, basically, whatever form that takes, but I've found lately, since the introduction of the NC, the amount of paperwork and administration required has increased and I'm spending more and more time doing administrative tasks rather than working with kids, which I think is the main priority of the job.

This point is evidently of concern to Sir Ron Dearing, who in his final report reviewing the National Curriculum and offering recommendations for its improvement, states: 'We must at all costs, avoid a complex, bureaucratic process which eats into teaching time and involves a great deal of administrative effort. Decisions to be made in the light of the present survey will need to give full weight to this issue' (Dearing 1994; para. 9.3).

However, in this study, teachers felt that the pressure they were under within the school day was enormous. It was creating a sense that no matter how hard working and how committed they were, at the end of the day they had achieved little. The demands of systematic assessment and record-keeping, combined with the generally conscientious approach of the majority of teachers, were tending to produce unreasonable and unmanageable work-loads, making the job of teaching intense and stressful (a finding supported by Campbell *et al.*'s 1993 study):

> I find that it is so very demanding the whole time, physically and mentally. If you are feeling under the weather or a little bit off, you cannot allow it to interfere because you cannot step back and just relax for a few minutes, which I think you could do in many other jobs. You have to be on top every time and I find it very, very difficult to have a

class as large as this and to keep them meaningfully occupied the whole time. I find that I work most evenings, come early in the morning and hardly get a dinnertime and it shows: by the end of term, I think I have used all my reserves. It is a very stressful kind of job, in a way, intensive.

. . . but the format with the files, folders and the attainment targets that we have to get to grips with as well. I suppose that has been an extra stress for teachers but, put that along with all the preparation that we are trying to do and all the extra work with new areas of study and the new emphasis on other areas of study, it really has become quite difficult the last two or three years, a lot more pressure, a lot more stress, a lot more physical work.

Thus, in addition to the first interest, teachers' second interest-at-hand, *workload*, was negatively affected. Under these circumstances it was not surprising that in each interview I had with teachers, the words 'no time' dominated their responses. Also every Monday, teachers' discussions within the staffroom were always about how dreadful and depressing this day of the week was, and every Friday they spoke about how exhausting the week had been. Teaching was becoming a quite unhealthy job. Further, taking into consideration that the majority of teachers were female (especially in the infants school, where this was true of all but one), a masculine business model in which work, not the family, has the prime claim on workers' time can damage female teachers' personal and social life (see Campbell *et al.* 1993).

The issue of workload is important in every occupation, but in teaching it becomes even more important as it is further associated with questions of commitment. Teachers' priorities were in conflict with the priorities imposed by governmental agencies; teachers emphasized 'real teaching' which prioritized time for planning and for being in contact with children, while the government emphasized 'service delivery' and accountability which prioritized time for assessing, recording and reporting results. This contradiction was perceived differently by different teachers, and feelings towards it varied in degree and intensity. However, teachers felt unanimously that devoting time to bureaucratic activities was influencing the quality of their job, as such activities were beginning to take over from teaching. Record-keeping was at the core of their dissatisfaction. Some teachers did not oppose the principle of keeping records because it was actually regarded as good practice and an activity they were already doing. They felt, though, that the reports were not accurate because there were so many of them:

We have to record what we have done. It sounds like a good idea but it's very hard to do for each individual child and for each subject. We have to make thousands and thousands and thousands of ticks in thousands and thousands of boxes that are all supposed to be accurate and, because of the size of the job, it's not accurate.

Others had strong feelings about record-keeping because they were confused about the nature of the particular records they were expected to keep.

The confusion of continual changes to the assessment and recording of results made teachers feel that such activities were purposeless: 'a waste of valuable time that should be devoted to teaching':

> In the National Curriculum you have to . . . well you're supposed to keep records of things that children have done and what level they've achieved and things like that [and] they keep on bringing out different sheets that you've got to fill in, so you're filling one in for a year or something and the next year they bring out one that they think is better, you know what I mean . . . Everybody seems to be producing their own. So each local education authority is producing what they think is the right one and the next year somebody else will produce a different one and it just gets too much . . . so in a way that tends to take valuable time up that you could be putting in to teaching.

For some teachers a factor which generated negative feelings towards the principle of record-keeping was the realization that it was not teaching, nor did it represent the reality of children's learning:

> The majority of her [the teacher's] work is intuitive and has nothing to do with pieces of paper, ticks, crosses and circles.

> Very often I find that a lot of the paperwork is a lie anyway, because you can say, particularly with children with moderate difficulties, you can say that this child has learnt this, and for that day [the child] might have, but tomorrow they know nothing about it and your job is to repeat and repeat, again and again. The paperwork doesn't justify the ends.

Despite the above feelings and opinions teachers spent a lot of energy and time in filling in the records. It is interesting that even though they found record-keeping hard to do ('I know from the bottom of my heart that nobody's going to take any notice of it anyway') they still devoted time to figure out what was the most appropriate way of 'twisting words', or of 'translating reality into jargon'. Probably this happened because 'of their training into an occupational culture in which a high value is placed on vocational commitment' (Campbell *et al.* 1993: 23). However, as shortage of time within the school day was one of the major problems for teachers, the issue of the 'presentation of the reports' was called into question.

Teachers' opposition to detailed formal record-keeping based on continuous judgement of children's progress focused more on its technical aspects than on the ensuing social consequences for children labelled 'different'. Even teachers who were opposed to the principle of systematic assessment and record-keeping did so on the basis of the confusion and technical impracticalities arising from its implementation, dubious validity and heavy workload. A possible explanation for this is that during the year that this study took place, the pace of change was such that the teachers' main concern was not the social patterns which would follow the new directives but simply the implementation of these directives. It was evident that some teachers were totally confused about the way the new system was supposed to operate:

> I couldn't tell you, to be honest. They [children with special educational needs] are meant to achieve within various levels but not having actually done the assessments, I don't know. I mean I don't understand half of it, well not even 10 per cent of it.

Even a Year 2 mainstream teacher who was directly involved in standardized assessment procedures for 7-year-old pupils, and was opposed to such testing, suggested that the testing procedures would eventually be abolished:

> We have this testing now that I don't feel is doing students any good at all. Most teachers know where their children are at, and yet we have to spend all this time on administrative work, administering and working out the tests, and, to me, a lot of that is a waste of my time, which I think could be spent in a more vital way. They are so young to be tested. I mean some of them had only five terms in school and we are already testing them . . . And the government places so much stress on them [tests], and the parents are getting worried. Everybody is getting uptight about them. It is something new that is coming. I think it would probably be abandoned in a few years because it is too early for them [children] to be tested, but we have to go through the process and suffer.

Teachers' cursory awareness of problems and consequences for children labelled 'different' was emphasized in Abbott *et al.*'s (1989) study: 'Clearly, vital equal opportunities issues are raised here but early findings on teacher implementation of assessment procedures from the PACE study do not show strong awareness' (in Pollard 1992: 114). Pollard goes further by stating that teachers had accepted the basic principles of teacher assessment probably because such teacher-controlled formative assessment was broadly consistent with child-centred philosophy and with the application of professional judgement. Responses such as 'I would say that all teachers are assessing children all the time, it's part of our professional responsibility' were not rare. However, three teachers, in particular, even though they did not express an opposition to the principle of teacher-controlled formative assessment, seemed to have strong feelings:

> Well I think the government by introducing the National Curriculum led parents to believe that standards weren't high. By introducing the National Curriculum and assessment at 7, 11, 14 and so on we would raise standards. I don't feel that's the case . . . To actually formalize [the assessment procedures,] that makes some sense but I think very little sense for children that have trouble with work [and] particularly when you then start talking about comparing results among children from school to school, that's nonsense. What I'm interested in is what each individual is achieving, where they come from and where the next stage is going to be.

You know that a school has to report on the performance of all pupils and I think schools are trying to be manoeuvred into competitive situations with other schools. So in terms of exam performance they have things like league tables so you can compare one school with another. I can see that some schools might be reluctant to take in children with special needs because they would not reflect well in the overall score [words missing] that are going to be presented to parents and the community at large. So special needs children don't really fit in well to competitive situations because in those terms they're not going to succeed.

I think it's [the publication of results] terrible, dreadful, irrelevant and anti-educational. It doesn't reflect the skill of the teachers because there are other factors [coming in to it, such as] the catchment area, the parental support which varies according to which part of the city you are in. So it's irrelevant and I am totally against it . . . I just think it's part of the political [words missing] of the current government, the Conservative government . . . Competition, free market competition and they try to apply that inappropriately to the educational system.

The emerging tendency (encouraged by the government) was that teachers and schools should be valued according to the published results of pupils' academic achievement; teachers were being pressurized to comply. A role strain arose for some teachers either because of the changes to the hierarchy of obligations dictating which expectation was to be accorded priority, or because they had to accomplish two roles that were not compatible: responding to children's needs by teaching accordingly, or responding to commercial/competitive needs by teaching towards the tests. It is useful to bear in mind that 'as long as teachers rely on examination results as the major proof of the ability to promote learning . . . preaching about developing the child's interests will have as much impact on the teacher's perspective as does a light breeze on the Tower of London' (Hargreaves 1972: 148). Some teachers – especially the ones who had adopted the more flexible child-centred ideologies – found themselves affected by a shift in the defining principles of professional commitment. Let us explore this further.

Throughout years of working with children, teachers in the study school had developed certain teaching styles which were based on their definitions of what constitutes teaching and learning, and had ascribed particular meanings to the notion of 'good practice'. In regard to teaching styles, it seemed that all but one teacher had, throughout the years of teaching, become more informal, more flexible and, because of accumulative experience, they had become more relaxed and confident. They had realized that teaching is a learning process in which changes take place according to the dynamics of the school, the dynamics of the class, the social elements that children bring to learning, and societal demands and expectations.

Some of the teachers, especially those with many years' experience, were aware they had changed their approach to teaching. They had started with fairly rigid and formal ideas about teaching, but in the light of experience they had realized that teaching is very complex and includes a variety of social functions. These teachers felt that under the new circumstances they had to 'turn back' to the more traditional ways of teaching:

> I think when I first started teaching I felt that it was my job to [convey] to children certain bodies of information, sort of what is a fact and knowledge, rather like I'm being asked to do now for the National Curriculum. But I think, as time went on, I realized that it wasn't my job to hand over great wadges of information, . . . so it [my approach] became more child-centred as time went on and now the National Curriculum is going back away from child-centred work, which is unfortunately very depressing.

> When I started you had to teach in a certain way . . . Now my approach is much more informal and it is geared much more to the children's needs. In the past, they were grouped according to their ability, now they are much more mixed, mixed abilities, mixed ages and there's much more individual work . . . [but] I think they are asking us to go backwards.

The essential point of contrast was not so much the emerging change of teaching styles but the values underlying what were perceived as 'progressive' and what were perceived as 'traditional' ways of teaching. This difference has been clearly identified by Rowland (in Bates and Rowland 1988), who argues that to subscribe to student-centred (or to subject-centred) learning is to affirm a set of values rather than to believe that a certain technique or set of techniques is the most efficient means of learning. The exploration of these values sheds light on the contrast between teachers' own conception of their role and the new political conception of it. The problem is that, like many basic concepts in the human sciences, the concept of role lacks any clear definition. However, Hargreaves (1972: 71) notes that 'role refers to prescriptions about the behaviour of a person occupying a given position, a set of guidelines which direct the behaviour of the role incumbent or the actor. Roles consist of sets of expectations.'

One of the basic guidelines influencing teachers' behaviour was that the social and personal elements that children bring into learning are of great significance, and thus must be involved in the structuring of learning and teaching activities. Teachers were aware that different children have different social histories, with consequences for learning. They were also aware that broader social trends are changing and that children are being affected by such trends:

> I think it's not only me who has changed but children have changed as well. They have much more knowledge, they travel a lot, they are interested more in general knowledge, they are more sophisticated. They are not more mature, they are not more grown up but they know much more. They are much more aware of the world around them, they have more stimulus from their environment, like the media.

Generally speaking we have these days a different type of problem to what we had when I was first teaching. Now, family relationships are different to what they were. There are a lot of children from homes where parents have been separated or been divorced and those are presenting a whole new range of problems that we did not have when I was first teaching.

Now family units are based mainly on both parents working. There used to be a great worry about having the key and going alone back to the house. It was a great worry for society because these children were on the street and today, even though it is still happening, people are not getting worried so much about it.

Teachers' awareness of wider social trends and the more specific social histories accompanying individual children tended to influence the way they perceived the functions of teaching:

There are a lot more problems with children [the new generations of children] that are coming in [to school]. There are many more family problems, emotional problems, behavioural and social problems that make our job harder, and we have to deal with them. I mean, if you are talking about teaching children, you cannot just teach them in isolation and impart knowledge. If you are talking about developing the whole child you have to take into account all the problems [and] it is getting harder and harder to do so.

Their perception of good practice included efforts to integrate the child's cognitive, social, personal and emotional development within the structure of teaching. This approach to education as a means of developing the 'whole' child rather than just parts (i.e. intellectual aspects) was associated with the structural characteristics of working within primary education (as compared to secondary).

Thus, they argued that at the core of teaching is the ability to contextualize learning. This involves making learning interesting, which presupposes the construction of activities which will attract and involve (in a meaningful way) the children in their classroom. This was of great concern as it affected not only children's experiences of schooling but their interests-at-hand as well. This, however, demanded not only being aware of children's needs but being involved in the creation of a curriculum flexible enough to respond to these needs, and appropriate under different circumstances. These ideas were vitally important to these primary school teachers and shaped their commitment and beliefs in educating children:

I've learned that there are no hard and fast rules. Each child is an individual and children respond to different people and different work in different ways and I think one of the skills of being a teacher is finding out what children enjoy. Yes, I'll use that word – *enjoy*. It's not a word you often hear in education but you have to find out ways in which children enjoy working, because I think if people enjoy what they're doing they will learn better . . . So I think there are no hard and fast rules and it's basically getting to know the child and what situation that child works best with.

Well, our approach is very child-based. We start off with children, the interest of the children in a particular class and you build your curriculum around those interests.

The term 'child-centred pedagogy' is quite abstract as an ideology and it can vary in the degree and nature of its implementation. Previous studies have suggested that, even though the Plowden Report was influential, fully developed child-centred practice was comparatively rare in classrooms because teachers dominated to a greater extent than envisaged by Plowden (Bennet 1976 and Galton *et al.* 1980, cited in Pollard 1992). Of course we have to be careful when using rigid dichotomies (such as child-centred versus subject-centred, progressive versus traditional, formal versus informal) in reflecting on teaching practices and styles in relation to effectiveness. As Hargreaves (1972: 75) notes, ' "traditional" and "progressive" are examples of the ill-defined labels we attach to different role conceptions within the teaching profession'. That happens because there are different role conceptions of teachers working within various segments of educational systems. Teaching styles do not match such dichotomies: they operate in more complex patterns (Berlak and Berlak 1981). Perhaps a more useful distinction is the one offered by Wolcott (1977) between teachers and technocrats. This distinguishes between those who focus on the development of the child (using traditional *or* progressive methods) and those who tend to serve dominant social groups by preparing students to be effective operatives within established systems of production. It seemed that teachers had to cope with a transformation which tended to favour technocracy.

Even previous to the introduction of the 1988 Educational Reform Act, it was evident that teachers invariably sought to control their students, direct their activities and were also occupied with teaching the basics of language and mathematics, together with other conventional areas of knowledge and skills (Delamont and Galton 1986; Hunt 1990; Pollard 1992). However, under the current climate, the nature of control (of both teaching and learning) seemed to be transformed as the following discussion indicates.

During the research interviews and conversations with the teachers in the study, it became clear that they held a view of 'good practice' that confirmed Pollard's argument, according to which

The Plowden Report encapsulated values which were vitally important to many primary school teachers in terms of their commitment and beliefs in children – the ideas of public service, of caring and nurturing, of responsiveness to need and of support for the disadvantaged . . . Such ideas formed an important part of the identity and sense of 'self' of many primary school teachers.

(Pollard 1992: 108)

Within this context, teachers claimed that an important part of their role was to identify and develop areas of interest around which the majority of children's work could be organized. This required not only the integration of subjects and space for negotiation, but also, most importantly, flexibility within the classroom, teachers' autonomy and involvement in creating the curriculum, a broad definition of the notion of learning and the provision of adequate time. The majority of teachers identified these elements as interdependent constituents of teaching and learning in primary education because their main concern was to match the curriculum with the diversity of children's learning patterns. These elements seemed to be the practical consequences of the more general philosophy of the 1960s and 70s concerning the aims of primary schooling. Pollard (1992: 106) summarized these aims thus: 'whilst there was an acceptance that education ought to equip children for the society into which they will grow up, a school was not seen merely as a teaching shop'. As a consequence, 'a hallmark of the effective curriculum was taken to be its flexibility and responsiveness to children's interests, a way of working which placed great faith in the professional judgement of teachers in its implementation' (p. 106). Teachers seemed to enjoy the faith shown in them even though they had to deal with a number of other parameters such as large size of classes, children with a wide range of cognitive, personal and social needs, and resource constraints.

In the current period of intense political and economic intervention, a shift in the aims of schooling is taking place whereby education is being made subject to market forces, and schools are being compelled to respond to external pressures and to reformulate their notions of children's needs. The job of educating children is viewed as central to the development of productive efficiency, and schools are in the process of becoming more effective in the development of human capital and in the production of commercially usable knowledge. One teacher viewed this situation in the following way:

> There's always a debate in education about whether we should be
> educating children so that they can perform well in their working life,
> economically, you know, teaching kids skills that they will need in their
> occupation and there is another group, another school of thought,
> which says, 'No, what we should be doing is educating children to be
> better human beings and to be more aware of the world and more
> environmentally aware, more tolerant of sexual differences and racial
> differences and we should be bringing children up in schools to be top-
> quality human beings'. My philosophy is both, not one or the other. We
> can do both. We can educate children for their job and for life. What's
> wrong with having clever, technologically skilled, scientifically aware,
> kind, honest, tolerant people? We can have both. But I believe that the
> wind is blowing strongly in one direction. We're being encouraged all
> the time to go for the first kind of person. I think the attitude coming
> from the government and the people who pay for our schools is more

and more that we should educate children for the economic good rather than the social good.

The emphasis on productive efficiency, as the main aim of the educational process, has had a number of consequences for teachers and teaching. One of these consequences has been the newly introduced educational centralism exemplified by the introduction of a National Curriculum. As two teachers strongly argue:

> The whole point of being a teacher is to decide what the children need to do, and now the NC is telling you what they have to do, so you don't need a teacher really, you just need a robot.

> I think the teacher who doesn't enjoy her work cannot do it. If you are a teacher and you just come in and say 'do this and that', you are not teaching anybody. You have to be interested. That's why there has been a big problem with morale in teachers.

Attempts at standardizing teaching in primary schools had a strong impact on some teachers' feelings towards the new political directives. This might have happened because previously, within primary schools, external constraints (such as uniformity imposed by the requirements of the syllabus of an external examination) had been rare. Teachers' autonomy meant that curriculum content varied greatly between different schools. Pollard (1992) has shown that the protection of autonomy was an important concern for teachers and constituted their third interest-at-hand.

In the new circumstances, teachers felt that they were losing autonomy. They now found themselves within a transformation in which the 'licensed autonomy' or the 'loosely regulated autonomy' (Williamson 1981) from direct state control that they had enjoyed in the past was becoming a 'tightly regulated autonomy'. The legislative imposition of the National Curriculum and the framework for its delivery represented a serious curtailment of teacher autonomy. This transformation brought further dissatisfaction:

> Up until about two or three years ago, until the introduction of the National Curriculum, what I particularly liked about teaching was the range and freedom of choice of the kinds of things you could do. So I particularly chose primary schools and middle schools because you were not restricted to syllabus in the same way that you are in a secondary school where you simply prepare for examinations. In a primary school there used to be much more freedom about what you did and how you did it. But now that's changed a lot because of the government's National Curriculum that has been imposed on schools. So some of the things I used to enjoy about teaching have now gone out of the window, have now been removed . . . now there is a great pressure, pressure on your time, there is no time to, sort of, pursue personal interests with the children.

I like working with children. You are fairly independent in what you
would like to do. Well, the National Curriculum spoiled that now.
That's why a lot of people have left.

In the new government-driven educational context, teachers were to be
blamed for declining standards while their professional judgement was under
assault from a number of misleading criticisms. For example, while the extent
of progressivism in teaching styles can now be seen to have been substantially
exaggerated, governmental agencies claimed that progressivism was rampant
(Hunt 1990). This argument was used, in a politically exploitative manner, as
the basis for centrally monitoring and controlling teachers and teaching.
Teachers were presented from different sectors of the media as being ineffec-
tive and non-professional. One of the aims of such criticism was to demoral-
ize and publicly disparage teachers and their professional judgements:

Teachers have been deprofessionalized. I think most teachers feel that
the media and the government have [words missing] that we've had so
much power taken away from us. We've had awful things said about us
and now we have to be told what to do . . . so I have very strong
feelings about the whole thing really.

I think parents have very much been led to believe that teachers don't
know what they are doing.

Some teachers revealed anger and frustration because of the criticism
directed at them from different quarters and because of the practices imposed
upon them:

I like to be able to teach, full stop, without having additional pressures
from the government, from the media, from people outside telling me
how to do things, that I am not doing them right, that I ought to
change it . . . I really feel that we are getting a lot of outsiders telling us
what to do, who are not involved actually in education at our level. I
really find that very hard indeed.

What really irritates me is all this crap that we are inundated with from
the government.

For other teachers, the new imposed directives were infuriating because

The people who live in these ivory towers who designed the NC they
have never been into a teaching situation or they may have been but
they have totally forgotten all about it because they have been divorced
from teaching and they don't understand what we are trying to do.

There were a number of reasons that led teachers to the creation of such perceptions.

The majority of teachers who participated in this study were not opposed
to the principle of having a national curriculum. Some teachers wanted a
national curriculum that would alleviate some of the difficulties of deciding

what shall be learned – a constant concern throughout their experience of teaching. They wanted guidance and a reference point that would enable them to reflect on their own practices and make sure that they offered breadth and balance:

> Personally speaking I've always found the part of the job that was most difficult was deciding what to teach and I was hoping that the National Curriculum would help me in deciding what to teach, but actually it made it many times worse.

> I think a good teacher will carry on teaching in exactly the same way as he or she always has done because children need teaching according to their own individual needs, not according to a curriculum that's been imposed from above for children who haven't got special needs. But I'm sure there are teachers, and I'm probably one of them, who would have benefited from a curriculum to the extent that it made us think about breadth, made us sure that we were not getting too concerned with reading or with numbers or whatever, that we are making sure that we incorporate computers or technology or geography or history at a very basic level.

From participant observations, it became evident that a lot of time, work and thought was devoted to the implementation of the curriculum. Teachers endeavoured to adjust their practices to the demands of the curriculum and vice versa. Throughout the process, however, they faced enormous difficulties in doing so, and a large number of concerns dominated their discussions in the staffroom and the interviews. The specific concerns varied from teacher to teacher, and different teachers focused on different aspects of the curriculum. Some teachers were more concerned with the prescriptive nature of the curriculum or the technical problems arising from the speed of its introduction and the communication of changes. Other teachers were more concerned with the lack of integration among the different subjects that they had to teach:

> In a primary school you tend to do, especially if they are young . . . you take something that is happening, let's say in autumn, so in autumn you have to cover some natural science, some ordinary science, some English, some maths, shapes, and all that will link together. Now, with the NC, each document has been done separately to all the others. I mean you can integrate them but it is much more difficult to do so. They never thought about linking it . . . It's not like secondary schools where you have to teach geography and you teach geography only, here we have to link work together.

This concern was expressed by a number of teachers who thought that both the content and the form of the National Curriculum had little bearing on the 'primary culture' and the learning characteristics of young children. They found it overwhelming, overambitious and hard to match with children's requirements. Some teachers, especially in the infants school, expressed the view that the curriculum was either 'irrelevant to the primary school context' or difficult to implement:

> I think that the primary level has hardly been considered. I think that a lot of the NC has been arranged from secondary aspects and it has just been pushed down to what they considered to be a primary level. We do feel that [with] a lot of the NC . . . I mean, they thought 'Oh what should they know when they will get to 16?'. They have done it and then they moved backwards from that. So they think 'OK, at the primary level, they should be doing this, this and this', and, really, I think it is of no relevance to children . . . Like in arts they [children] have to study other painters and recognize other painters by the time they are at 7. It seems hopelessly wrong to me. Lots of children in 7 just draw a face and things like that and to have to recognize somebody's masterpiece . . . oh I think it's so ridiculous.

> Sometimes, the areas of the curriculum that I think pose the most problems are things like, arts, PE [physical education] and technology. The way it is written down, it's very difficult to interpret and to find something appropriate for the children to do.

> There is certain work that must be done, that must be covered. Now we are halfway through and I think we managed to keep up, luckily. We managed to get some of this extra work done but I know I have Christmas coming up. We have Christmas plays and cards to make and decorate classrooms. Well, it has not been considered, in the NC, all the work that has to be done before Christmas.

In addition, teachers commented that there were curricular requirements that reinforced a restrictive notion of learning (including the transmission of vast amounts of information), promoted an idealized image of children, and lacked flexibility. These bore little resemblance to primary teachers' view of learning:

> You cannot do things . . . You cannot repeat things, and going over and over. You need to do this with kids; but you don't have time to get back. Their [the creators of the National Curriculum] idea is that once you've covered it, it's there for good. Well it isn't. It needs reinforcing. It needs going over and over and over but you just don't have the time to do that. That sort of thing irritates me. There are, in every class, two or three [children] who are able more or less to keep up with everything as the curriculum sets it out, but that leaves all the rest to often hang in a complete flounder because you just don't have time to do it in the depth that they need to have it done. So in the end, you gonna end up with . . . them knowing less because you can't cover it in a sufficient depth . . . It is ludicrous.

> Like, for instance, Peter. He cannot fit in anything like that. He cannot

fit into the class. We cannot teach him like that. He needs flexibility within the class and the NC does not allow much flexibility. Children like Peter, they need to develop ideas that they've come up with. So if Peter is interested in something and he needs to work in the work he's interested in, now, if you work on that he will learn. If he had to follow the NC he would have to do so much work each day that most of it will just turn him off.

Matching the curriculum with the children's diversity, which for the teachers in this study was the core aspect of teaching, had become even more difficult to accomplish:

The biggest difficulty is matching the work to the individual's needs, the individual's abilities, because we always teach mixed-ability classes so you get a big spectrum of ability. It is important to produce work that is suitable and matches the abilities for this range of children and that's the biggest single challenge; because if you don't get it right you get all types of problems and anxieties from the children.

This difficulty is of a high concern to teachers because keeping their classes in order by occupying children in a meaningful way reflects their ability of 'being good at the job'. This is their 'best defence against criticisms which could adversely affect teacher autonomy . . . Being good at the job is also a means of satisfying other concerns such as obtaining enjoyment and managing stress and workload, and it also relates to gaining the respect of colleagues' (Pollard 1992: 28). In other words their performance in class influences their self- and professional image; consequently teachers could be expected to disapprove of whatever constraints endanger their image of 'being a competent teacher'.

In summary, the above discussion has focused on the way teachers perceived the conditions within which they had to work. This includes the way they felt that their interests-at-hand (such as satisfaction, workload and autonomy) had been affected by the newly introduced political directives. The overriding message communicated by teachers was that of personal dissatisfaction, frustration and anger about the constraints within which they had to work. For the majority of teachers, teaching did not give the same degree of enjoyment and fulfilment that they had experienced in the past, because they felt compelled to fulfil different and conflicting expectations. Maintaining their principles, values and standards they believed in had become a complicated process, creating tension and extreme physical and mental fatigue. They were profoundly affected by a shift in the defining principles of professional commitment.

The recent economic and political changes and their cumulative impact were having a negative effect upon teachers' morale and motivation. These two elements are highly significant under the current circumstances in which teachers felt that they had to intensify their efforts so as to preserve a balance between the demands of political and market forces and the demands of children. Such demands are difficult to reconcile.

The teachers interviewed, however, despite their expressed dissatisfaction, were still in the profession. Presumably to secure the continuity and survival of their approach to teaching they will partially comply with and adapt to the new circumstances, even though the type, mode and nature of that compliance will vary from teacher to teacher. The teachers' quality of being 'adaptable' and the ability to be 'sensitive' to the environment within which they have to work help teachers to accommodate and retain a sense of professional identity. In turn, the formation of teachers' professional identities is being influenced from the different kinds of cultures of teaching. These teaching cultures 'comprise beliefs, values, habits and assumed ways of doing things among communities of teachers who have to deal with similar demands and constraints over many years. Cultures of teaching help give meaning, support and identity to teachers and their work' (Hargreaves 1994: 164).

The educational activity can be seen as a dialectical interplay between structural/situational constraints and teachers' ideological commitments. This interplay is similar to what has been called the 'overlap' between the teacher context and the educational context (for an extended analysis of these two terms see Keddie 1971 and Pollard 1992). Within the *teacher context*, the emphasis is on the teacher's routine, the daily contact with pupils within the classroom and all the practical activities that surround it. This is the highly pragmatic world, the world of 'is' rather than 'ought to be' (Keddie 1971). It includes teachers' perspectives on what is or is not possible in given circumstances, and teachers' strategies and techniques for achieving goals (Pollard 1992). This context influences and is influenced by what has been called the *educational context*, which is represented by commitment, idealism and a continuous effort to implement equality of educational provision (Pollard 1992). The educational context includes paradigmatic strategic orientations, and views about 'how things would be in an ideal world'. Thus these two contexts are not mutually exclusive. In fact, they overlap, and one affects the other in the teachers' everyday world. The assumption underlying such a view is that individuals are not 'taken over' by cultures. They can both contribute towards and be influenced by them in a dialectical process (Woods 1983). In this sense teachers can become policy-makers within their environment, a role that attributes to them power and responsibilities. There has been a growing realization that

> The teacher is the ultimate key to educational change and school improvement . . . Teachers don't merely deliver the curriculum. They develop, define it and interpret it too. It is what teachers think, what teachers believe and what teachers do at the level of the classroom that ultimately shapes the kind of learning that young people get.
>
> (Hargreaves 1994: ix)

I will go on to use this idea of dialectical interplay to focus on the process of integration with specific reference to children with Down's Syndrome. However, before embarking upon capturing and presenting teachers' attitudes towards the integration of students with Down's Syndrome, some clarifications are necessary. A main theoretical (methodological) principle underlying the majority of conventional attitudinal studies is the importance of the specificity of the attitude referent group. This has been highlighted by Gottlieb and Siperstein's argument, according to which,

> People who are mentally retarded [*sic*] vary greatly on any number of characteristics that could influence attitudes towards them. A valid appraisal of attitudes towards mentally retarded [*sic*] persons, therefore is dependent on a precise description of the population that is the focus of the attitude expressions. Accordingly, a recent review of the literature indicated that a primary reason why the attitude data cannot be easily synthesized in a meaningful fashion has been the failure of investigators to describe precisely the referent about whom subjects are asked to express their attitudes . . . In circumstances where no descriptive information is provided, it is difficult to determine subjects' conceptions of a mentally retarded [*sic*] person; consequently their attitude expressions are difficult to interpret.
>
> (Gottlieb and Siperstein 1976: 376)

This is not the principle underpinning reference to children with Down's Syndrome in this study, because such a research/ideological principle perpetuates a number of disablist assumptions. First, it implies that the impairment of the individual is the ultimate source for generating attitudes, with little reference to the social contexts within which attitudes have been developed in the first place. Thus it decontextualizes attitudes as being apolitical, asocial and ahistorical (see Chapter 2). Second, by using the disabled person as the main reference point in exploring attitudes we focus, unreflectingly, on only one side of the disability relationship – the disabled person – with little reference to the behaviour, roles and perceptions of 'the others' as representatives of a socially determined disability relationship (Finkelstein 1980). Third, such a principle perpetuates the dominant tendency to explore the attitudes that people hold towards the individual who has an impairment, with little or no reference to the social restrictions which are imposed on the individual. Finally, by implying that the problem resides within disabled children/people we promote a certain conceptualization of the problem which hinders attempts towards the creation of an alternative way of both thinking about and acting on issues of disability.

As Finkelstein (1980: 6) argues, 'Whether one sees attitudes as being associated with something in the individual (the impairment) or with the social situation has a profound influence on how one interprets the results of research.' The starting point of analysing and interpreting the material gathered from the fieldwork was the exploration of the practices and ideologies that hindered or promoted the creation of inclusive education. From this perspective, teachers' expressed attitudes towards the integration process served as a means of identifying institutionalized ideologies and practices within which certain attitudes have been developed. Thus, the expression of attitudes was perceived as a social phenomenon, a 'communicative act', which is context-specific and culture-bounded (see Chapter 2). In efforts to clarify why teachers were responding in certain ways, it became evident that discussions about teachers' meanings and feelings towards integration could not be separated from their understanding of educational policies, the practices of schools as institutions, and teachers' attitudes towards the notion of difference/disability.

Within this context the rationale of using children with Down's Syndrome as a referent group initially was created out of the complexity and the nature of stereotypes embraced in expressed attitudes towards these children (see Rynders *et al.* 1980; Booth and Statham 1982; Booth 1985; Buckley 1985; Morss 1985; Stratford 1985). As Tony Booth argues,

> People with Down's Syndrome are subjected to two sets of prejudices; those concerned with their distinctive appearance and those about their relative incompetence. Theories of racial degeneration have been linked to the perception by some that they look 'Mongolian'. They have been barred from schools because they look 'handicapped'. They have all been viewed as severely mentally handicapped despite a wide spread of abilities, and insofar as they have been regarded as mentally handicapped, they have been prey to all the prejudices that attach to that label too.
> (Booth 1985: 3)

However, throughout the fieldwork and during the process of analysing teacher's responses, it was evident that integration is a complex notion, regardless of who was to be integrated. The complexities involved within integrational practices and ideologies often influenced teachers' attitudes towards this process, whether they were referring to a child with Down's Syndrome or to a child with dyslexia. Some common patterns, concerns and principles applied to the integration of all the children with special educational needs educated at the school. For this reason, the discussion in the following chapter unfolds mainly around the issue of teachers' attitudes towards integration while, whenever necessary, there is a particular reference to children with Down's Syndrome.

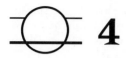 **4**

Teachers' attitudes towards integration (with reference to pupils with Down's Syndrome)

To begin with I will focus on the way teachers define the notion of integration. This will offer us a starting point for discussion because definitions allow for the creation of a dialogue and offer an ideological framework within which people make sense of cultural, social and political phenomena (see Chapter 1).

The school has approximately 350 pupils. For the last seven years an integration policy had been implemented by the creation of an 'integrated resource' which catered for 40 students with special educational needs. According to the school's official prospectus,

> The school has an integrated resource for children with moderate learning difficulties. Children come into the Resource on a Statement of Special Needs. The aim is to enable children to live and work with children from mainstream school. They will be found therefore, in any classroom working with the class teacher supported by a member of the Resource staff or one-to-one with the Resource Staff or in a small withdrawal group. Occasionally children are totally unsupported in the mainstream classroom. Whole school involvement, teaching and staff (teaching and non-teaching) are part of an educational process whereby the acceptance of these children in school leads to their acceptance in society as a whole.

Integration, officially, was perceived as an educational process which will enable children with moderate learning difficulties to live and work with their peers. The stated ultimate aim was integration in the wider community. Teachers' responses, however, suggested that integration both as an idea and as a practice had no shared common meaning. It rather meant different things to different teachers, and often it meant different things to the same teacher:

> To me integration means many different things and it means different things for different children, so I don't really think we can have a blanket rule and say 'this is integration'.

In the main, teachers offered a definition of integration that placed 'special needs children' in a different pedagogical category, who could only be incorporated within ordinary classrooms on condition that they could cope with established educational routines. From this perspective, teachers were looking at the application of integration within an educational environment without questioning the terms of pedagogy which would involve changing teaching practices to make curriculum content more accessible to all children:

> I like to see them [children with special educational needs] in the class working with other children at their level, doing basically what the mainstream students are doing as much as possible. Now really that would mean that they weren't on a group of their own, that they would be actually sitting with mainstream children doing similar work. But I find that by this age the gap is too wide for them to be integrated for most academic situations.

> [The way I understand integration is] that the children with special needs are fitted in with those who are normal, and are able to mix and work with mainstream students side by side. There are certain times that you have to withdraw them for certain things, but it's nice to see them in a classroom. It's just acceptable.

For other teachers, integration had a wider definition associated not only with the microcosm of primary school but also the macrocosm of wider society. The following responses reveal how complicated the idea of integration was, especially when continuity did not exist. Further, as the following examples illustrate, 'for teachers, what goes on inside the classroom is closely related to what goes on outside it' (Hargreaves 1994: ix).

> Real integration should take place with children in the neighbourhood schools – to go to their local schools, so that the child plays with children in their road, goes to school with them, is educated alongside them, goes home at the end of the day. Certainly with our children they have a dual role, they have different friends out of school than in school.

> Children are being integrated at a younger age and then it breaks down at secondary level. I don't think it should break down. I think the danger is that people won't adapt, the kids have got to fit the system, not the system fit the kids.

> Integration? Well, I would like to know what happens to, how can I say, our kids when they leave secondary school. Because at one time there used to be placements across the city for them to go for work experience and things like that. Now I believe they are closed down and I just don't know what happens to them. So it seems to me a lot of hard work that has been put in during the school years is suddenly just dropped and finished with and the kids are then out in a wider society and they've got no aid, no support and they are very much left to their

own devices . . . As far as I know I think I've taught probably, perhaps 35 kids and as far as I know only two have got jobs, which is worrying isn't it?

Other teachers, influenced by the constraints within which they had to implement integration, were quite suspicious about 'the real motives' underlying the movement of integration as presented by governmental agencies:

> It was presented to us that these children would gain from being integrated with the mainstream children, both socially and academically . . . It was claimed to be the answer to all sorts of problems, the way forward and all that. But the cynical side of me says that it is just a method of cutting costs. You know it is cheaper to put them all into one building . . . If it's been done genuinely to try and integrate them into society as a whole, then it is a good thing and you know it should continue. But I suspect the motives of the people in power are different than the ones they claim.

> I think that it [integration] will eventually end . . . Now the trend is to get more and more children in, and we are always under threat because of financial pressures and I think all the time being pressured to increase the number of children we have and I know they'd like to reduce the amount of teachers that we get to deal with these children . . . You get even more children to a school like this and then what are you doing? You put them in a separate room? . . . If Patroklos [a support teacher] was looking after these children in a separate room he'll probably look after eight or nine, so you can get more children into a normal school and call it integration but the only time they are going to be integrated would be at play time. So they can close all these special schools down and put the children in ordinary schools but, without back-up, you can only put them in their own group – you know, put more kids in which is cheaper.

Teachers' visions of integration (that could be implemented in an ideal world) were interfering with 'realities' which were constraining not only from a materialistic but from an ideological point of view as well.

It is important to note that teachers' attitudes towards and understanding of integration were anything but clear-cut. The material obtained from the fieldwork was very rich in meaning and insight but at the same time extremely conflicting and confusing. In dealing with the tensions and conflicts I encountered in making sense of teachers' responses, I was helped by Apple's (1993) analysis of the politics of common-sense, in which he explains how elements of ideologies of groups in dominance become truly popular. A central point of Apple's (1993) work is the importance of connecting our analysis with the real life-experiences of the people under investigation. This proposition was crucial in understanding teachers' conflicts and confusion surrounding their perceptions and actions towards inclusive practices. This is especially so in an era where ideas of civil equality are being shaped by market forces.

According to official claims, the introduction of the National Curriculum and subsequent directives promotes the entitlement of children with special educational needs to a broad and balanced curriculum. However, such assumptions ignore that 'policies tend to present directions which are couched in unproblematical terms with little indication that they are compromises between many sets of ideas, needs and interests' (Mousley *et al.* 1993: 60). They also ignore that major social changes in both attitudes to disability and pedagogical practises are necessary if praiseworthy rhetoric is to become reality. Exploring teachers' attitudes is extremely significant because 'the teacher is the ultimate key to educational change and school improvement' (Hargreaves 1994: ix); s/he is in the forefront of implementing stated policies within constructed educational realities. As Mousley *et al.* (1993: 59) have stated, 'it is difficult to develop policies which define "what will be" without careful consideration of "what is" in terms of history, beliefs and attitudes'.

In light of the above I propose to analyse teachers' attitudes towards integration from the perspective of curriculum design. As Apple says,

> I do not approach the issue of curriculum design as a technical problem to be solved by the application of rationalized models . . . rather . . . I conceive of curriculum as a complicated and continual process of environmental design. Thus do not think of curriculum as a 'thing', as a syllabus or a course of study. Instead, think of it as a symbolic, material and human environment that is ongoingly reconstructed. This process of design involves not only the technical, but the aesthetic, ethical, and political if it is to be fully responsive at both the social and personal levels.
>
> (Apple 1993: 144)

Within this symbolic, material and human environment the way teachers identify different children is of great importance because it shapes how they interpret and interact with the pupils that surround them. The understanding of differences in achievement and classification of pupils has been submerged in the routines of teachers' work and thoughts, and frequently there is no call for teachers to articulate it (Carrier 1990). However, teachers offered extensive explanations and clarifications of what they meant by 'children with special educational needs' in their definitions of integration. Teachers focused heavily on the individual child in order to justify the amount, the quality and the nature of integration that was taking place. So, among other things, integration was strongly presented as being about 'resource children'. The contradictions and different sets of expectations implied in the recent concept 'resource children' affected teachers' attitudes towards integration. In turn, the cultural understanding of this term was shaped by a number of institutionalized – including structural, personal, ideological and material – constraints.

Defining and responding to 'resource children': institutionalized influences

Within the infants school there was a separate room called the 'resource room'. This was the place where children with special educational needs were educated when both support and mainstream teachers decided, for a variety of reasons, to withdraw children from ordinary classes. Four support teachers (two of them part-time), called resource staff, were attached to the resource; their main responsibility was the education and the care of the 'resource children'. From participant observations it was noted that children with special educational needs spent almost half of their day in the resource room.

The junior level did not have a separate resource room. Instead, there were a couple of free rooms which were accessible to all students in case activities had to take place outside the main classrooms. The general idea was that the five support teachers (two of them part-time) could occasionally use these rooms when they felt that the children had to be taken out into smaller groups to pursue academic or other activities. From the perspective of physical integration it was noted that in the junior level less withdrawal took place than in the infants.

According to both mainstream and support teachers at both the infant and junior level, the general philosophy behind integration was that they should support and educate children with special educational needs *as much as possible* within mainstream classrooms:

> The philosophy was that, as far as possible, we would support children in mainstream classrooms. So we started off on the basis that all the children are part of the mainstream class, that they are on a mainstream class register, they are in such and such a body's class rather than in the unit or in the resource . . . We started working from the mainstream classroom that the child belongs to.

However, while in one class, children were educated for almost the whole day within an ordinary class, working with or mainly alongside their peers, in another class children were mainly withdrawn for the major part of the day and in a further class children were withdrawn only when the teaching of specific subjects was taking place within the ordinary class. This variation indicated that what was considered 'to be possible' varied from teacher to teacher:

> I think that it [integration] never intended that children should go into the classroom all the time.

> The idea [of integration] is that if they are in this class they are no different from anybody else. If they [children with special educational needs] are in my class, they are my class and I would do everything I can to help every child. So if Spyros [a child with Down's Syndrome] is in my class, then he is just like everybody else. He's got his own problems, his own worries and it's up to me to try and get over those.

> I would have them integrated in such things as games, PE, music, art
> and I would remove them from the room for maths, English, science,
> history, geography – the more academic things.

Even though the above responses indicate that teachers' ideologies and commitment influenced at least the amount of time that children were to be educated within ordinary classes, teachers themselves claimed that the amount,
the nature and the quality of integration was contingent upon the characteristics exhibited by different individual children. According to all the teachers,
one of the main criteria of defining what was considered possible and beneficial lay in some inherent characteristic of the child:

> Now in my class there are six of them and I think only two of these six,
> who are what I call true moderate learning difficulties, can gain
> something. The other four are quite severe learning difficulties and
> there are at least two of them who, you know, have a lot of other
> problems. They gain nothing from being mixed in with the rest of the
> class for everything. But the problem is that it's thought to be ideal for
> them to be integrated for everything, which I do not agree with.

Teachers' responses revealed that too much of integration relied on children's
personalities. They found that lately more children with special educational
needs, with more and complex difficulties, were being integrated into ordinary school. The majority of them, especially mainstream teachers, tended to
dislike what they saw as a 'trend' of integrating children just for the sake of
integration, a trend that ignored the added complications for teachers.

Some of them thought that an ordinary school was not the appropriate
place for some children with special educational needs to be educated. One
teacher had developed a polemic stance towards 'the new fashion of integration' and, as he bluntly put it, 'you've got to be really really insane before
they will actually put you in a separate school'. Such attitudes were based partially on teachers' beliefs that some children with special educational needs
(especially students with Down's Syndrome), due to their 'deficiencies' could
not be educated together with mainstream children.

One of the core pedagogical assumptions which seemed to remain
unchanged was the focus on individual children in justifying exclusive practices. Often many teachers used phrases from the government policy documents, such as 'whenever that is appropriate for them [children]', in defining
educational practices. At the same time, however, such a focus seemed to
clash revealingly with actual policies-in-use.

The official school document stated that 'the school has an integrated
resource for children with moderate learning difficulties'. Teachers had
accepted this description as being necessary for obtaining resources that
would enable children to be educated within the school. However, tensions
arose in their effort to understand where exactly the distinction should come
between every pupil's own special needs and the special educational needs of

a 'sizeable minority' group of children called 'resource children'. Teachers' confusion and tension in defining the terms 'moderate learning difficulties' and 'special needs children' (which were used interchangeably) reflected the influence of the ambiguity and non-specific nature of the Warnock definition of 'special needs' (which has been incorporated in both the 1988 and 1993 Acts). A support teacher found it hard to define integration because he was puzzled with the notion of 'moderate learning difficulties':

> I think there's always been a problem defining what is a moderate learning difficulties child. Still I've not come across a satisfactory definition. I believe that all children have got learning difficulties. I mean all children, all people have got needs whatever they may be. I find it very difficult to define and to categorize some needs as special. I mean, those needs and those difficulties change with time and with situations. That doesn't make anything any easier. That makes the situation more complex and more difficult to understand.

A mainstream teacher thought that by differentiating and overemphasizing some needs as special, justice was not done to the rest of the children whose needs were ignored. It seemed, however, that under the pressure of structural constraints she had accepted this 'ordinary injustice' as forming an element of the established pedagogy:

> I've got children in the mainstream that have got difficulties of their own, and I would like them to have a bit more time and attention that the support teachers are able to give to the special children. I know that my poorer mainstream children would benefit so much if I was able to give them more of my time or if another teacher was able to give them more time. They would benefit so much and yet they cannot have it [time or attention]. They just have to have only one teacher for all of them. *I regret that but that is how it is.* [emphasis added]

Teachers trying to specify the ambiguous term 'special needs' created a number of categories. First, children with special educational needs were differentiated by the rest of the children and were referred to as the 'special children' (as the above quotation illustrates). The reduction of some children to a bureaucratic entity in this way became its own justification for treating the members of this category as a separate group. Within this group, children were further categorized as 'special needs children in terms of behavioural problems', 'special needs children in terms of emotional problems', and 'special needs children in terms of "genuine" learning difficulties'. However, this further categorization did not solve any of the complexities encountered, not only because different children did not fit into such painstakingly made categories but because different teachers had different and contradictory perceptions about the same children, as the following responses illustrate:

> I think the biggest concern is this: I think first of all the definition of a child with learning difficulties is important. I know that the children

who come here are not special needs children in terms of behaviour. Now if we're having special needs children with behavioural problems that would be totally different, a totally different kettle of fish. I don't think it would have worked nearly so successfully.

Well I think that if they were all genuine moderate difficulties, in other words they were just academically slower than the other kids then, yes, I think that they [children with special educational needs] would gain from being with the mainstream children. But so many of the kids that come through here, supposedly just moderate learning difficulties, are in fact behavioural problems and have got any other sort of problem as well.

One way of explaining the above contradiction has been offered by Mercer and Richardson (1975), who pointed out that 'handicap' is a cultural category which implies that those identifiable as 'handicapped' will vary according to people's cultural orientation. This suggests that there is a potential for confusion and conflict when people try to talk about a so-called 'handicapped' person. It also suggests that the range of possible outcomes for integrated children was influenced by the way they were perceived by different teachers. At this point it is relevant to note that some teachers held a negative attitude towards the integration of children with Down's Syndrome because these children, according to teachers' perceptions, did not fit within the definitions they had ascribed to the term 'moderate learning difficulty':

I know some of the staff think that none of the Down's children should be in. Under the definition of our unit, I don't think they should have been in because I think that mainly the other children could fit more accurately to our unit. You see with our definition of the unit we expected moderate learning difficulties.

The majority of teachers strongly appealed to the within-the-child difficulties (as we shall see) in justifying their views. It was often forgotten that children were evaluated on the basis of whether or not they could fit into pre-specified definitions, which were highly influenced by institutional demands and practicalities. The following responses illustrate some of the institutional demands that had influenced the construction of the 'resource unit' in the first place:

Well, you have to take responsibility for seeing children before they come to the resource. Seeing if they're of a level that fits into our criteria.

I think given that we haven't got enough resources and we haven't got the staff, we have to choose the children very carefully to make sure that they are children that can cope with this sort of integration.

Downstairs [at the infant level] we have four staff so having them [children with special educational needs] in four classes it is common sense that they will either be supported or withdrawn. If you have them in five classes somebody will have to do without support which is not possible . . . We may have a lot of children in one particular year group, we may have none in another year group, so we have to sort of balance out how many we can cope with, within each class. Also if they did move up [to the junior level] perhaps they wouldn't have room in the classes upstairs. We have to juggle with numbers ourselves otherwise it can be very overburdening. Like perhaps in the downstairs department we may have 20 per cent of the children and upstairs they may have 80 per cent of the children, which wouldn't work. [So some children with special educational needs did not move upstairs on a specific year because of these constraints.]

A selection process was taking place as to which children could be integrated within the school. That process was mainly based on whether or not the children could fit into what the school could or could not offer. Teachers claimed that selection and right placement were among the most difficult, complicated, and extremely important processes:

The process of placing and moving children is so complex. I think that the placement of the children is so critical, it's really the basis for the whole integration.

In cases where problems arose due to 'wrongly placed' children, the source of the difficulties was to be examined only from the perspective of material resources. Thus children were becoming the scapegoat of a complicated situation:

We had children who were wrongly placed because we could not meet what they required. We haven't got support . . . If you get a child who perhaps has been wrongly placed or finds it difficult to come to terms in being in a mainstream situation it is very very hard to cope. Everything seems to revolve around this child, and one child who perhaps is being particularly difficult to integrate can actually upset the whole feeling of the class, which may be in itself a difficult class. So integration can fall down because if you have one child who perhaps has more difficulties it means that you have to withdraw more which is not fair to the other group of special needs children who also have to be withdrawn as well.

Selection, placement and resources were among the major concerns of teachers. These concerns were amplified as more and more was added on to existing structures and responsibilities of their job. Simultaneously, little was taken away and still less was restructured to fit the new expectations of and demands upon teaching children with special educational needs. The fiscal crisis made it nearly impossible for the school to have sufficient resources – especially in the infants school – to meet all of the goals they were expected to meet. Teachers' decisions and children's education were heavily predetermined, which made the process of integration more complicated and reinforced the development of resistance to the inclusion of children with special educational needs in ordinary classes.

> When we were to have the Resource in the school we were promised a lot of things that never really came. It did sound that the staffing was going to be really very very good. We were also told that we were going to have smaller classes so that the special needs could be integrated into a small class. But when you are getting classes up to nearly 30 plus the special needs children it [integration] falls down really.

> But I would not want too many of them [children with Down's Syndrome] at once. I think one or two each time is enough to be integrated in the class because there are the other unit children as well, and it is very tiring. I have so many other children with difficulties and behavioural problems and policies do not help.

> The main problem is that we don't have a lot of cover, we don't have a lot of staff. If we got the staff we'd be all right but you see downstairs we are running the 20-place resource on 1.5 teachers and 1.6 support. What can they do? I mean, in terms of quality with the children. You can work it out but there is no quality and the children are very young, they need support. I don't think it's fair for the children and for the staff . . . Sometimes they are integrated on sight not integrated in the classroom.

From the perspective of support teachers:

> I think there's going to be some kind of reaction from mainstream colleagues who are going to say 'We cannot cope' or 'We do not want these children in our classes anymore.' I feel that is starting to happen already . . . so that's one concern.

> I mean quite rightly most mainstream teachers feel they've got a difficult enough job, particularly with the National Curriculum and everything, without having to think about special needs children as well. I can see why they might actually resent the children being in the class. I can see why these children are being viewed as an extra burden.

Given that pedagogical structures had not changed towards the direction of inclusion, the focus was on whether children could fit or not. Given that the focus on the within-the-child difficulties had become an internalized form of pedagogy, teachers' orientation was leaning towards modifying children's characteristics. Such a point of view emphasizes parts of the child and belittles the importance of seeing the whole person within a social situation. Thus teachers revealed two major concerns in regard to integration that were associated with within-the-child characteristics: their behavioural difficulties and their cognitive disabilities. A further exploration of these two concerns can shed light on how institutionalized structures influenced and shaped teachers' attitudes towards integration.

One part of the child: behaviour in context

It was indicated above that different teachers had different perceptions of the same children. At this point, however, I would like to stress that children's behaviour seemed to be of a high concern and that the majority of teachers associated the notion of 'special needs' with the existence of behavioural problems, even though they were aware that some mainstream children exhibited greater behavioural difficulties than some of the children with special educational needs. The association was so strong that 'special needs children' in teachers' perceptions implied 'behavioural difficulties' even in cases where teachers did not have any actual encounters with specific children. This association was even stronger when children with Down's Syndrome were concerned. Teachers' resistance into including 'resource children' in ordinary classes for the whole day was based on the argument that children needed a lot of individual attention and a lot of one-to-one contact due to their 'unpredictable' and 'disruptive' behaviour. Children's behaviour was a key issue in discussions about integration:

> They ['resource children'] are disruptive to everybody else and so neither side [mainstream and 'resource children'] gains. I think if they can be separated out and their behaviour sorted out, if that can be sorted out, and can be modified then it's fair enough to be mixed with, you know, ordinary kids.

> If they have learning difficulties they can integrate probably better but the children that have behavioural difficulties as well as intellectual difficulties, they need so much individual attention.

> One of the main difficulties of implementing integration is their behaviour and this depends very much on the individual child.

From this perspective, children's behaviour was the key determinant of the amount, quality and nature of their inclusion within ordinary classes. Several points need to be noted. First, teachers' strong association between learning difficulties and uncontrolled/uninhibited behaviour was no surprise. For example, many people associate learning disability with erratic and uncontrolled behaviour, with instability, unreliability, and even cruelty and violence (Carrier 1990). This association can be explained by referring to the historical development of special education, its sociopolitical aims and public perception (see Chapter 1). Second, it indicates that initial encounters between a teacher and a child with special educational needs did not start from a neutral point. Prejudices about children with special educational needs had already been constructed previously and independently of any encounters with these children, and had been highly influenced by the negative social connotations that the term 'special needs' implied:

> I'd no experience with children with special needs . . . when the boss [head teacher] said we were going to have an establishment of a 40-place resource in our school . . . and it would be called an integrated

resource with children working as far as possible in a normal classroom, I thought that it was going to be a disaster.

The association between 'special needs' and 'uncontrolled behaviour' was a part of broader well-established social assumptions which tended to be more negative in relation to children with Down's Syndrome. The existence of such preconceptions was evident in teachers' responses about how they felt when they were first called to teach children with Down's Syndrome:

> I didn't have any experience [of children with Down's Syndrome]. I was very apprehensive. I didn't know whether I was able to teach them because they seemed as though they would be awkward and not cooperative. They looked like they were not going to be cooperative with the teacher. But I was pleasantly surprised really after establishing a relationship with them.

> I never had Down's children before. They were the first ones I came across . . . I was quite apprehensive before they came into my class. I have heard all the stories of Spyros. He was the first one I had in the class, and I've heard of how naughty he could be when he wanted to be a naughty boy, and I thought 'Oh dear'.

Teachers' view of children with Down's Syndrome were based mainly on pre-assumptions of what the children could not do; this had influenced teachers' initial encounters with these children. This can partially explain why teachers were initially reluctant to agree to include and educate children with Down's Syndrome. However, teachers seemed to associate 'resource children with attention behavioural difficulties' for a number of other reasons closely related to the educational activity. I would not like to imply that children's actual behaviour is of no concern – but focusing solely on children's behaviour does not take us very far because behaviour has meaning only in relation to the way teachers perceive and evaluate it. Mehan *et al.* (1986: 80) has clearly shown that 'instead of attending to behaviour in isolation, teachers are attending to action in context'.

The way teachers perceived different children's behaviour has to be viewed within the traditional educational pattern: that of typification and categorization. Of course, the process of typification is a broader life phenomenon in which human beings understand things by naming them; thus to name, categorize and label things and/or persons is an inherent part of understanding them (Hargreaves *et al.* 1975). It has been found that typologies are used by teachers to help them operationalize definitions of the situation and simplify the educational activity (Woods 1977, 1986; Pollard 1992). Teachers build their expectations upon such typologies, which become stereotypifying social categorizations. These seem to be fundamental to teaching practices because teachers act upon and respond to each student accordingly.

In turn, the process of typification and categorization (as well as teachers' concern and focus on the behaviour of children with special educational needs) has to be viewed in a wider context, and as part of a more general traditional concern: that of keeping order within a classroom. It was noted (from participant observations) that teachers were highly concerned about minimizing the sources of disruption and often used different mechanisms to do so. Because the disciplinarian subrole was so central a task in classrooms, pupils' behaviour which threatened this role was perceived negatively by teachers and was either discouraged or even punished – in the case of children with special educational needs often withdrawal from the classroom was used.

In every class observed, teachers felt that they must be in control. To be in control means that

> The teacher must be able to make the rules of conduct and obtain conformity to these rules by the pupils. When the teacher is either unable to impose rules and/or attain obedience to them, s/he is said to have failed in his/her disciplinarian role, for the pupils are out of control or undisciplined – masters of the situation.
>
> (Hargreaves 1972: 144)

Rules were applied to all children including children with special educational needs. As a mainstream teacher put it, 'they [children with special educational needs] need to know that what we [teachers] say is what we expect to happen'.

Keeping order, maintaining the rules and fostering obedience had become an inherent characteristic of the educational activity. It was noted that teachers devoted a lot of time in negotiating disciplinarian tasks with their children. Participant observations confirmed Pollard's argument that

> Teaching the children and 'keeping them under control' are not undertaken just because that is what teachers are committed to doing or are expected to do: they are also undertaken because it helps the teachers to 'survive' and defend their concerns in the classroom.
>
> (Pollard 1992: 34)

Of course teachers' personalities, the way they perceived their subrole as disciplinarians and the way they resolved discipline tasks differed from teacher to teacher, affecting the organization of their class and in turn affecting the nature of integration.

However, daily educational activity was based on certain routines that mainstream teachers expected children to go along with. Most of these routines, including the rules applied, were taken for granted as self-evident and indispensable in promoting educational activity. Children had to conform to these routines whether they accepted them or not. Different educational routines encompassed different sets of expectations. Children were expected to conform and 'behave properly'; teachers defined what was 'proper', which was different in different contexts. The same routines and expectations applied to all sorts of children, including children with special educational needs. Whenever children with special educational needs did not conform to these routines, the tendency was to judge the child's behaviour and to assume that to be able to conform was a beneficial social skill:

> They have to adapt to our mainstream routine and this is a real advantage, instead of being sheltered in a special school where everything would have been catered for them.

> Well, there are a lot of social benefits really. They have role models. They are learning a lot. Clair, for example, she is in Mrs O'Neill's routine most of the day. She does not always understand, when she is sitting on the carpet, what is going on, I mean, not always, but she copies the other children. She is learning to conform.

Conforming to the rules, and copying 'good models of behaviour', was viewed as a social benefit because in teachers' perceptions it was associated with raising expectations for these children. It was a social skill to be learned for coping with life. Learning to live within the wider community meant, in teachers' perceptions, learning to conform to the rules and imposed realities. However, support teachers especially were more aware that children with special educational needs had to conform within an educational reality where the 'whole timetable is geared to the mainstream children'. Support teachers, working closely with children with special educational needs and trying to respond to their dynamics, were more understanding than mainstream teachers when children did not conform to the established educational routines. They were aware that the routines which children were asked to cope with were not designed with them in mind. Thus support teachers, in explaining why some children exhibited 'disruptive' behaviour, instead of focusing on the child, often referred to the curriculum and its inherent expectations. Support teachers seemed to act as mediators between children with special educational needs and mainstream teachers, a role that caused some tensions:

> Sometimes you feel pressure because you feel that a lot is expected from the children and that is difficult for them. You want to protect them from that and yet they've got to get used to relating to the mainstream teacher and do as they're told. It's not easy for them because we are asking a lot of them. You have got to make them behave for the mainstream teacher and then at times you feel that you can quite understand why they are not always conforming. But you have to keep them conforming because you don't want to upset the mainstream teacher. Your job is to see that your children are conforming . . . Quite a lot is expected from them but then again they have to learn something living in this world.

> Well, I fear that there are a lot of problems for the mainstream teacher . . . I mean, I can understand why special needs children can be disruptive in the middle of the story. It must be hard for them to be expected to listen to the teacher talking to the mainstream children or reading a story which does not correspond to their level. They find it quite difficult to listen and the teacher finds it difficult to pick up the pieces and continue.

We have enormous expectations of them in terms of conforming and at times we can understand why they do not conform.

Further, other support teachers' explanations why children's behaviour was targeted and defined as 'disruptive' referred not to the behaviour itself but to teachers' attitudes towards teaching:

> I suppose certain teachers would not want them [children with special educational needs] in their classrooms because they [teachers] use certain carryings on and they don't want to be disrupted because occasionally you can be disrupted by one of our children . . . I think it takes a lot more work and it is very much harder [to teach special needs children within ordinary classes] but, if you can get it to work, it is very fulfilling and it depends on the teacher, basically, if she is a good enough teacher to be able to cope with all the different things.

> Well, inevitably when you have these children in the class you get a higher level of noise certainly because they find it difficult to do certain things . . . [and] if they are sitting next to the other children even if you give instructions the noise rises . . . But it depends very much on the attitude of the [mainstream] teacher . . . I mean different teachers have different ways of working. This year I find it very enjoyable to work with Carol [mainstream teacher] because she is cooperative, we share ideas . . . she doesn't mind so much about the level of noise . . . Last year I found it difficult to work with Roy because of his way of working . . . he found it difficult to interact with another adult and he couldn't cope with the certain amount of noise that you inevitably have to cope with when you have these children in the class.

Most of the support teachers indicated that one of their roles was to facilitate the disciplinarian role of mainstream teachers, even though at the same time they realized that in doing so too many changes were expected from children with special educational needs. At the same time, however, support teachers, from their interaction with mainstream teachers, had realized why some mainstream teachers tended not to be able or not to want to cope with behaviour that did not respond to the rules imposed within ordinary classes. The observations by the two support teachers quoted above suggested that mainstream teachers' attitudes and abilities 'to cope with all the different things' were key determinants in promoting or hindering inclusive education. However, the tendency of mainstream teachers to focus on the child's behavioural difficulties in justifying exclusive practices has to be viewed within the wider context within which the teachers had to work.

Under these circumstances it seemed that teachers could hardly cope with any type of behavioural disruption. On the one hand, teachers had to deal with large classes of 30 children. There was a wide range of abilities in each class. Every class included children from two year-groups; one class, for instance, had Year 3 and Year 4 children. This type of classroom composition demanded the provision of more diversified programmes and had implications in terms of classroom discipline. Let's listen to a teacher's voice in describing her experience of teaching a mixed-ability class of 31 children:

> It can be very difficult. I have to plan 31 individual programmes but because this is impossible I do work in groups. We have five groups so I am planning for five different areas and levels . . . Planning should be very, very carefully thought through. The basic thing to remember is that everybody has got some strengths somewhere and that you've got to sort of work on those. You have to praise children for what they can do, and then give them the confidence to do things that they can't. The less able children do need so much time and that's where the frustration comes in because there is so much you could do and you know it, but you cannot do it with the numbers that we have in a class. You need extra help because in a class of 30 it can be very difficult to share your time because the children at the top end of the spectrum need a lot of help in furthering their education. It's not right to assume that they will just go on. They need direct teaching as well as the less able children. It can be very hard not only in planning the work that they are going to do but in planning the teacher's effectiveness with each different group or even with different sorts of children. It is very weary, very tiring, because there is such a terrific regime amongst the children.

Even for such a teacher, who found it 'challenging' and 'rewarding' to teach children with a wide variety of abilities, being in a mixed-ability class of 31 children was difficult and tiring.

In addition to the demands stemming from mixed-ability classes, teachers had to deal with a number of complicated social issues that children brought into school. As we have already noted in Chapter 3, increasing numbers of children were coming into school with more and more social problems, different to and more complex than the ones teachers had to deal with 20 years ago.

On the other hand, as Chapter 3 indicates, teachers' work had become increasingly intensified, with teachers expected to respond to greater pressures. Pressures derived from four main sources: first, the government drive for accountability which had raised expectations and required more record-filling and paperwork; second, demands for 'raising standards' and the implementation of a centrally regulated curriculum which, according to teachers, was 'ridiculously confusing', 'overambitious', and perceived children as mechanical absorbers of vast amounts of information; third, the tendency to separate the social from the academic aspects of learning; and fourth, fiscal constraints. All of these pressures tended to produce extremely long working hours. Comments such as 'It seems you have to do so many things within so little time', 'You don't have time', 'It is a very stressful kind of job, very intensive', ' I come early in the morning, I work most evenings, and I hardly get a dinner time', 'My job has been made many multiples more difficult', were among the most frequent comments teachers made during the research interviews and in staffroom discussions. With such a workload, teachers came under an enormous amount of stress in their efforts to fulfil their increasing obligations. Such working conditions had a great influence on their willingness and ability to cope with demands deriving from inclusive educational priorities. The teachers' priority tended to be 'how they could best manage their time' while at the same time responding to what they felt were their obligations towards the children. As a consequence, mainstream teachers often claimed that they could not cope with 'resource children's' behaviour and that they were transferring the responsibility of educating 'resource children' to the support teachers, claiming that their priority was the education of ordinary children. Including 'resource children' in ordinary practices was viewed by some teachers as an 'extra burden'; 'resource children's' behaviour was used as one of the reasons why these children could not be educated together with their peers. This practice was justified by the teachers' fear of spending too much time with 'resource pupils' to the detriment of other children in the class:

> If they [children with special educational needs] start to become important you feel that the mainstream children are losing and that is when I find it really difficult.

> If they [resource children] are not taking it [attention or time] from the special teacher or whoever is with them they are demanding it from the mainstream teacher and that is where you feel 'Oh, my dear'. I have the mainstream children and, you know, a lot of them, they have special needs, they need so much help, and you have 30 of those children and then you have to deal with the others as well. I mean, there is the time involved when they [resource children] need you and you don't have time . . . [but also] there is the physical thing, because you get tired. You try to devote so much of your time and energy to the mainstream children and there are so many things to do with them that you really cannot afford the surplus energy that needs to go to the special needs children.

> They [mainstream children] get a lot of work in a short period of time. It is difficult. We have to cover more things now and that means we cannot get into some things, so you skip over things quickly. You have to do only one lesson about something instead of doing three or four lessons. So somebody like Peter [a child with Down's Syndrome] who is causing distraction has to be withdrawn because if the class is going to be distracted in this one lesson they are missing out. There is no chance to repeat things again and again.

Some mainstream teachers had to work hard in accomplishing what they felt were their obligations, often feeling guilty at not being able to do so. Guilt is a key notion here. As Hargreaves (1994: 142) so powerfully reminds us, 'guilt is a central emotional preoccupation for teachers . . . [However,] while guilt is a deep personal trouble for many teachers it should also be remembered that within many of our personal troubles reside compelling public issues. In his analysis Hargreaves associates guilt with the way the work of teaching is organized and structured. Exploring the different strategies teachers adopt to deal with, deny or repair this guilt, he suggests that

> Teacher behaviour that is excessively guilt-ridden and guilt-driven can become unproductive and unprofessional . . . In many cases, teachers' behaviour can degenerate into exit, burnout, cynicism and other negative responses as they attempt to cope with the intolerable burdens of guilt that are imposed from without and that evolve within.
>
> (Hargreaves 1994: 150)

One such guilt-driven opinion expressed by some mainstream teachers was that 'if children [with special educational needs] start to become important you feel that the mainstream children are losing'. Such reactions – arising from the intensification of the job of teaching – were making the commitment to inclusive education more difficult to maintain.

Within these structures, children with special educational needs were in danger of experiencing a higher degree of differentiation. The above complexities were further exacerbated by a strong deficit-medical approach of perceiving 'resource children'. Even in cases where teachers saw themselves as being committed to integration and held positive views about the benefits deriving from inclusive practices, they seemed to have been influenced by the well-established and popular medico-psychological approach to children. The exploration of the teachers' second concern – with another 'part' of the child, that of his/her cognitive disabilities – is revealing in terms of 'how ideas arising from the practices of "special education" were being imposed on the integration process, limiting teachers' visions of educational opportunity for all' (Mousley *et al.* 1993: 59). The reinforcement and perpetuation of such ideologies can be explained only in relation to the ordinary institutionalized educational practices within which integrational practices had to be developed.

Another part of the child: cognitive disability and 'specialization' within context

In addition to the behavioural characteristics of the child, a further determinant of possible outcomes from integration for each individual child was the way teachers perceived his/her academic abilities/disabilities. It seemed, as Sharp and Green (1976: 21) have suggested, that even 'the notion of child-directed learning is related to the categorisation of the pupils via the control problems presented to the teacher in an open fluid context'. It has already been mentioned that teachers' biggest concern was to match the curriculum with the wide diversity in learning patterns shown by children, because it affected the performance of their second sub-role: that of being an instructor. The way teachers performed this role influenced the way they performed the disciplinarian role and vice versa. Each teacher interpreted and performed this role differently according to their personality, background, training, attitudes and needs. However, a common pattern was revealed in the language used by the majority of teachers in referring to children with special educational needs. Often the common usage name of the child was replaced by a medical/psychological or even a bureaucratic label. It was used not to depict one aspect of the person's body or skills but to define their whole personality. Expressions such as 'Down's children', 'moderate learning difficulties children', 'resource children', 'dyslexic children' and so on were among the most common labels used. Language was dominated by the deficit medical model to such a degree that often within research interviews the word 'children' was omitted. Thus children were 'the specials', 'the special needs', 'the Down's', and 'the moderate learning difficulties'. Most of the previous transcriptions are representative of this dominant tendency. The following are some further examples:

Ryan Frixon: an MLD with a great many problems . . .

Peter Palmer: an MLD, Down's Syndrome, needing a lot of help, working in one-to-one in class with all sorts of problems . . .

Sara Russell: a dyslexic child who cannot put words down, with great many problems in spelling . . .

The language most teachers used in describing a situation or a child seemed to be in contradiction to their perception of being positively orientated towards integration. The following responses come from two teachers who had commented positively about integration:

I don't think it is, I am going to be very provocative at this point, I do not think that anybody in the right mind thinks that special needs children can come into mainstream, do everything that the mainstream children do in a modified curriculum, even that, I think is pie in the sky because the work is not suitable. I mean we were always taught, when I was in college that the work should fit the aptitude of the child and it should always be in context with the child and the context of an MLD is not the context of a mainstream child. You've got a child who is 8 years old functioning at $3\frac{1}{2}$ years old. How can you expect even in your wildest dreams that you can take the child into mainstream and modify the work so much. That child, and I don't say that for every time, but even with the work being so modified, how could it be in context with that child? Not even in your wildest imagination; the child is not ready for that situation.

If you ask me whether they are benefiting at the moment I would say two of them are and the third isn't, because he's not ready for it. Well, at least I think that's why he's not benefiting. I think two of them are benefiting enormously because they've got reasonable social skills and an awareness of what's going on and so are actually learning from the other children. Whereas the third one is too delayed really, has got very little language and hasn't really got the social skills.

This approach to children tended to reinforce teachers' perceptions that in order to facilitate the process of integration they needed support from special teachers who often were assumed to have extra knowledge and skills:

> You need a teacher who specializes in special needs children . . . who is able and qualified to work with them.

> I know that kids with special needs can't succeed in a normal classroom except with very special support.

> You've got to have adequate and specialized staffing; that is the main thing.

On first sight it might be argued that lack of special training was a reason for mainstream teachers to feel insecure about their involvement in teaching children with special educational needs. Indeed, as the above responses indicate, some teachers presented this as being the case. This can be understandable, as the popular image has been that specialized qualifications are important in dealing with the children in question. As Mousley *et al.* (1993: 66) note, 'even teacher training institutions continue, through the provision of "special settings" and "appropriate" professional courses to imply that these children have educational requirements which cannot be met by ordinary classroom teachers'. Within this context the principle that good teaching practice is good for every child regardless of levels of ability tends to be forgotten. However, there is another side to this story.

The teachers in this study were aware of what constitutes 'good practice' but, under the conditions they had to work they could not cope with facilitating 'good practice for *all* children'. Exploring their responses further, it became evident that they needed support from 'special teachers' not because they felt professionally incompetent to teach children with special educational needs but because the intensification of their job meant they needed another adult in the class to help them with what they were expected to accomplish. Support (specialized) teachers were indispensable, not due to their specialization, but because they alleviated the mainstream teachers' workload. In this case, the argument for specialization was used by mainstream teachers as a reason for obtaining support, and by support teachers as a reason for enhancing their status and justifying their professional existence. The following responses indicate that support teachers were indispensable to integration because of the practical help they offered to mainstream teachers in reducing some of their workload. In some cases, support teachers were there to withdraw potentially 'disruptive' students or deal with them in such a way as to ensure the smooth functioning of the ordinary system:

> There must be someone to remove the resource children and get them out and let the mainstream teacher and children go on.

> You need another teacher, really, who can work with them because the range is too much for one teacher to cover realistically within such large classes.

I wouldn't like to do it [integration] by myself. It would have been impossible. You cannot do it by yourself . . . I cannot imagine myself doing it without support . . . if you have another teacher then it is easy to happen and if there is a distraction [from children with special educational needs] the other teacher can take the child out and work out the situation.

It [the existence of support teachers] is absolutely essential, unless there is an activity like story time which, if they do not have behavioural difficulties, they can be in and then I am supporting them as well.

The specialization argument was also used to justify and enhance the status of support teachers' work. The following responses, even though they present different aspects and concerns of the way some support teachers perceived their role and position, are indicative of the nature and status of their job:

We are, if you like, guests and that works in various ways, depending upon the mainstream teachers' expectations.

I always feel like a guest in the classroom. I always feel that I've got to be aware that our children . . . the [mainstream] teachers are very good with them, I don't say anything that, er, . . . but I feel that I am a guest in the classroom and I have got to give back all the time . . . I don't like the children to disrupt the rest of the class. I always feel that I have to do extra things to make up for the privilege of our children being in the classroom. [Mainstream] teachers are very good but I do give them back a lot as well.

I also think that the mainstream teachers want a lot of training on what we [support teachers] are trying to do because I don't think the mainstream teachers understand what we are trying to do.

The career structure for teachers within an integrated resource is very difficult. You are, at the moment, neither a special school teacher nor a mainstream school teacher. You fall between the two and, in terms of moving on or looking for promotion, people are never quite sure where to move on to. I think that has implications in that people are coming into integrated resources, perhaps as a great commitment to integration, but where does their career take them then? The salaries aren't the same as working in a special school. Colleagues here, if they were working with the same children in a special school, would be on an allowance for doing so. They don't get that allowance, nor do mainstream teachers get any enhanced allowance for having these children in their classes.

From all the above responses, it seems that the same ideologies and concerns employed a hundred years ago for the development of special education were being used currently in referring to the development of 'integrated resources'. These findings support Mousley *et al.*'s (1993: 61) argument according to which 'integration had become very much a resource issue and teachers demanded retention and extension of those very factors which characterize special schooling – withdrawal areas, training of teachers in specific responses to different categories of children and comprehensive resourcing based on assumed needs'.

Given that little had been restructured to meet the demands of teaching children with special educational needs, integration was still perceived from a materialistic (resources and staffing) perspective. Such an understandably strong preoccupation made it difficult to look at pedagogical issues. Additionally, the emphasis on resources and extra support staff further differentiated resource children from their mainstream peers. One support teacher expressed concern about the current tendency of referring and labelling children, who could previously cope in ordinary classes, for the purposes of proving a need for extra support:

> I think teachers, because of the pressures that they've got in a class of perhaps 30 students, understandably – I am not criticizing mainstream teachers at all, but children who traditionally in the past might have gone through a mainstream school and eventually succeeded – I think now there is going to be a great temptation to say 'This child isn't achieving. I'm spending an enormous amount of time with this child and I cannot afford that. Therefore, we'll have to statement him and find out where he is at.' The statement is being used to get the children some extra help. Now that's not wrong in itself. I am not saying that the statementing procedure is wrong. What I'm saying is I think that the knock-on effect of the National Curriculum and the pressure it puts teachers under will be that more and more children are statemented, perhaps at a very early age. I think there had been a tendency in the past in this school to say 'We will give this child a chance. We will try. We will make allowances for the fact that this child had a lot of absences through ill health. We will perhaps make allowances for the background initially.' Now I think the tendency is to say 'This child is difficult. We will start statementing procedures' because, you see, that takes a long time in itself and special educational needs is almost becoming a growth industry.

The above teacher was concerned that an increasing number of children were going to become 'resource children', not solely because of the difficulties that they presented in teaching but because mainstream teachers, under the new working pressures, will resist offering children a second chance. Furthermore, the process of differentiating some children and focusing solely on 'deficiencies' had become such a strong institutionalized practice that it both shaped consciousness and was reinforced through the patterns and routines of everyday life. Some teachers had internalized and accepted, as a self-evident truth, that some children were 'resource children' mainly because they had 'special needs' and vice versa; an assumption which made it difficult to explore the reasons why they were deemed to be 'resource children' in the first place.

The overwhelming majority of teachers in this study tended to treat educational difficulties as brute facts, as 'natural objects'. From this perspective, according to some teachers, children had to be or were already in the 'resource unit' because of their inherent characteristics hidden beneath the surface of their actions. Further, teachers' responses indicated that the process of integration was associated with the process of normalization. The process of normalization, however, has two distinct meanings. The first implies normalizing people; the emphasis is on meeting established expectations and modifying aspects of the individual child. According to this view, integration becomes a mechanism for making children conform to models of perceived normality, or at its best, is concerned with finding a way of encouraging and educating people, teachers and children to accept and tolerate those who deviate from normality. The second meaning implies questioning the concept of normality, valuing difference and understanding that a person becomes devalued not through his/her 'differentness' but through negatively valued 'differentness', which is contingent upon other cultural and social factors. According to this view, integration is not only about tolerance and acceptance but about rights and an endeavour to integrate differences (see Chapter 1).

Normalization within the process of integration

The notion of difference was extremely important for teachers in the study because (a) it was a source of contradictions and conflicting perceptions, and (b) it seemed to influence the angle from which they viewed the benefits of integration. It seemed that teachers often vacillated between an ideology of valuing difference, a liberal humanist ideology of accepting and tolerating difference, and a practical perception which demanded conformity. The notion of difference had both a positive and a negative connotation.

Teachers seemed to perceive children with special educational needs as different from mainstream children. Simultaneously, however, teachers claimed that they endeavoured to treat children with special educational needs in the same way as the other children so that they would not be viewed by their peers as being different. The aim of these practices was to encourage ordinary children to accept and tolerate children with special educational needs (the two words 'acceptance' and 'tolerance' were often used interchangeably). The majority of teachers strongly believed that one of the benefits (if not the main benefit) of integration for mainstream children was to learn that there were different groups of people in society and they had to accept these people as being 'normal'. Thus valuing difference meant accepting, tolerating, empathizing and sympathizing with people who are different:

> It's a massive advantage I think for the ordinary children in the
> classroom because they see that children with special needs are not
> physically different to them and when they [ordinary children] get out
> into society I am sure they'll have more sympathy, more empathy and

treat the children with special needs, when they [ordinary children] are adults in a different way, in a better way than if those [children with special educational needs] had been isolated away from them in a special school. They don't regard them as oddities or objects of fun . . . they are remarkably tolerant and kind.

They [mainstream children] are going to grow up with these children and they are not going to think that people are freaks because they are different. They are going to treat them as normal people which they are . . . Our mainstream children are very good with them. They have quite a lot of patience. They know that they [children with special educational needs] are different, but they are all very kind to them, they are quite tolerant.

One teacher was strongly orientated towards educating children to be kind and tolerant as this ideology was strongly reinforced by his religious commitment:

Well, I am a committed Christian and I went to church on Sunday and the preacher was telling a story about Saint John who when he was in his nineties was still preaching. They used to have to carry him up into the pulpit so that he could preach to the congregation. Every week he only used to say one thing, he used to say 'Brothers and sisters, love one another', and then he'd sit down. And the people in the church kept saying 'Well, we're going to all this trouble to lift you up into the pulpit, carry you up there and every week you say the same thing: "Brothers and sisters, love one another." What about all the complicated things in life?' And Saint John said 'Well what else is there to Christianity? Love one another, that's all it is. That's it, there isn't any more, forget everything else just love one another.' That's deep in my heart and basically I try to spread that by example, without being soft about it. Tolerance, love, kindness. I don't want those things to disappear from our society. I've an awful feeling they've been pushed out of our society and been replaced by selfishness and greed so I am trying my best to encourage kindness and tolerance.

One teacher seemed to be clear about the distinction between valued and devalued difference; instead of talking about tolerance, acceptance and sympathy she associated the notion of valuing difference with rights:

I think that for those children who are going to be able to go on and lead a fairly independent life that it is extremely important that they grow up with 'normal' children around them so that hopefully they don't grow up feeling 'I am different and I am not wanted', they grow up feeling 'Yes I might be different but I am wanted, I am part of a wider group and I'm valued for who I am.' I think the school certainly has a role to play in terms of educating mainstream children that our [support teachers'] children, yes, might be different but they still are people who've got rights, who have got abilities as well as disabilities and who are members of this society.

For other teachers to be different meant 'not being normal', even though there was a sense of guilt in using the word 'normal':

I think it's wonderful for the parents when the child comes into, I shouldn't say normal school, I know we shouldn't but we do. But sometimes it might give parents a false illusion that one day their children will be normal.

According to this perspective it was a matter of privilege and not a matter of rights for children with special educational needs to be educated in ordinary schools: 'I always do extra things to make up for the privilege of our children being in the classroom.'

Finally, according to another teacher's point of view, being different meant 'not being as fortunate':

Basically [the main benefit of integration for the mainstream children is to realize] that everybody is not as fortunate as they are. I mean, the main thing is to see that they are more fortunate than the other children. I don't think they understand at this age why they are more fortunate. I don't think that they internalize the fact that the resource children are brain damaged. I don't think that they appreciate the complexities but, it seems, they see that there are people who are not as fortunate as they are.

From teachers' responses it was indicated that there was an overriding attachment to normality: normality seemed to be an attribute that existed and could be defined. The underlying assumption, that was taken for granted, was that everybody wishes to be normal. Being different, according to this point of view, had a negative connotation and was viewed as an unwanted attribute, which had to be tolerated and at best accepted. Children were valued not on the basis of their difference, and of who they were, but rather on their efforts to become the same as the majority of the other children: to become 'as normal as possible' or to be viewed as 'normal'. Some teachers felt that their obligation was to treat all children as being the same, even though they were aware that different children had different needs and talents:

They [the specials, according to the teacher's terminology] do watch how the children behave, and they do copy a lot. I think that the acceptance they [the specials] usually get from the other children is wonderful. To be accepted as a normal person not as somebody special, as somebody different. I think that is very important.

I think that this is how they [children with special educational needs] see it. That they need a bit more help . . . At this age, they do not feel that they are different or we do not treat them as different. We try to make them feel that they are the same as the other children.

I, as much as possible, treat them [children with special educational needs] the same as [I treat] the others [ordinary children].

Clarifying the meaning teachers attributed to the term 'same' is difficult. There is always the possibility that teachers used the word 'the same' as a synonym of the word 'equal', even though 'equal' does not mean 'the same'. The majority of teachers did claim that they treated children with special educational needs the same as they treated mainstream pupils; however, that was not the case in practice. In practice, there was a distinction between 'the ordinary/normal' children and 'the specials', ordinary classrooms and resource units, special schools and normal schools, 'our [support teachers'] children' and 'their [mainstream teachers'] children'.

The effect of the National Curriculum on the education of children with special educational needs: the teachers' perspective

Chapter 3 has already shown how teachers felt and thought about the National Curriculum in its wider context within primary education. Teachers found it hard to implement the National Curriculum because (a) it had little relevance to the practicalities of the circumstances in which they had to work, (b) it bore little resemblance to their views of teaching and learning, and (c) it was overambitious in regard to the amounts of knowledge that children had to and could absorb.

Each teacher was further asked to talk about the benefits derived from the National Curriculum for the education of children with special educational needs within ordinary schools. Teachers expressed different feelings towards different aspects of the curriculum, and the majority of them focused on concerns rather than benefits. In regard to benefits, only one mainstream teacher speculated that the National Curriculum would ensure that children with special educational needs would experience a wider range and depth of curriculum areas than they had experienced previously:

I suppose for children with special needs, they too will now be exposed to a larger range of curriculum areas so that might be the case, I think that would be a benefit. But to be honest, I haven't thought about this in depth for special needs children because I don't actually teach any in my class.

One of the support teachers claimed that the National Curriculum offered structure to learning while two other (support) teachers felt that the requirements of 'teaching by objectives' had been a well-accepted and established practice in the area of 'special education'. However, the majority of teachers, both support and mainstream, strongly suggested that the requirements of the National Curriculum bore no relevance to the needs and demands of learning for these children:

Personally speaking I can't see any benefits for our children because the National Curriculum does not take into account that our children are working and operating on different levels.

Children need teaching according to their own individual needs not according to a curriculum that has been imposed from above for children who haven't got special needs.

They [integration and the National Curriculum] just do not come together at all. It is farcical to expect that special needs kids could begin to cope with the NC as it stands. When you reckon that special needs children are given an extra six months to catch up and (I think, I'm not sure about this, but I think) they'll have to go through the same tests as the other children, oh, this is ridiculous.

I do not think it [the National Curriculum] is going to be relevant to children with special needs. There are areas like history, technology, geography that really have no relevance at all to children who have difficulties. I mean, even for the mainstream children. It is not relevant to them at this stage. We have children who cannot write their names and so to talk about history and geography when they are not in the stage of reading and writing their names is ridiculous. I think it is totally irrelevant. So for children with special needs I think it is even more so.

The emphasis on predefined developmental levels strengthened the ideology of the 'within-the-child difficulties' and magnified the gap between what 'resource' children could not achieve in relation to their mainstream peers:

Some students [with special educational needs] are not able to work at the first level . . . The children working at the early levels are usually children in infant schools but our children [with special educational needs] are in junior schools and they're still not attaining those levels . . . Some of our children do attain Level 1 and Level 2 but we're talking about children of 8, 9, 10 attaining levels which 5- and 6-year-old ordinary children attain.

Coupled with this, the pressures imposed on teachers by the demands of accountability to parents put most of them under enormous stress. Teachers were especially concerned about the negative consequences that the National Curriculum, with its testing, might have on their relationship with the parents of children with special educational needs, as following responses illustrate:

Well, really when I am testing them they all have to take a 'W' which means that they're all working towards something. But even so, I do not think that the special needs will really get much further than 'working towards' for years and years. So really the tests are not relevant to special needs children but they are doing it . . . It is stressful for the parents. I mean, they [governmental agencies] introduced this idea that children at 7 years old should be doing this, this and this, and that they should be getting to Level 2 etc. I think, that [it] will put the parents under a great deal of stress and anxiety, if they see that their child is not even getting to Level 1. I'm afraid that they could not understand that we are working to their child's ability, not to what the government thinks they should be doing.

If I've got a child who's operating on a language level of eighteen months old, how can I possibly teach him something which is appropriate to a 5-year-old with a 5-year-old's level of language? So the National Curriculum has not been thought through properly . . . Instead of putting a child in a position of having to be working towards the first level all the time, I prefer to say that the National Curriculum isn't appropriate for them.

I think it can do a lot of damage . . . I think particularly for parents who read about the National Curriculum and feel their children should be following what the curriculum has set out . . . It would be hard to explain to them that the curriculum isn't right for their children. I mean there are a lot of children with special needs who will never reach the first level of the National Curriculum right through their whole school career. They will always be working towards Level 1 of the National Curriculum. I feel that no child should be in that situation. I think for those children it would be better if there wasn't a National Curriculum which forces them to work towards it all the time and never gets them anywhere.

It's very difficult. If you keep saying to a parent 'your child can attain Level 1 in the National Curriculum', what happens the year after when they are still only attaining Level 1? It looks to people as though they've not achieved anything within that year or within their whole school career. But what they're [people] actually missing are the laborious steps that you have to take to achieve certain levels.

Parents have heard this thing about the National Curriculum, but they don't actually know what's included in it and so for the parents of the children who have got special needs it becomes even more difficult to understand, 'Why are they [their children] never improving in any way?'. But you see the children *are moving somewhere* but as things are, it's difficult to appreciate it.

Parents see what a child at 7 should be doing and they would like to know why their child at 7 isn't achieving that . . . Now what we've [teachers] got to do is rejoice in the progress that the child has made and say 'This child has made absolutely enormous progress. He's still functioning at this level but he is great. This is what the child has to do next, this is what he could do when he came into school.' I think we have got to have a very positive attitude towards our children.

The above responses illustrate some of the consequences derived from the newly introduced curriculum scheme where children had to be evaluated against predefined levels, which bore little relevance to their development and way of learning. Pressures for accountability may force teachers to focus on the within-the-child difficulties in explaining why some children fail in a system that provides 'a legal entitlement of all pupils to a broad and balanced curriculum'.

It was noted above that most mainstream teachers were committed to striving to bring out the best in every child, but that did not mean that all of them wanted or could work with *all* the children, including the 'resource children', under the current circumstances. However, given that these children were educated within this ordinary school, the pattern observed was that they had become second-priority children for some mainstream teachers and the main priority for support teachers. This allocation meant that mainstream teachers could maintain a supportive veneer while taking the minimum responsibility for educating these children:

> Well I don't see a lot of their academic work. They come and show it to me occasionally and I usually praise them but I must admit it is in a superficial way because I have to do so many things with the other [children].

Children with special educational needs were mainly included in activities such as PE, music, story time, craft, art, and in the infants school, playtime. In most of the other circumstances 'resource children' were either withdrawn from class or were working as a small group with their own task and their own teacher, alongside, but not together with, their peers. However, from participant observations in three classes it was noted that all three mainstream teachers (with the help of the support teachers) were integrating what they called 'activity days' within the curriculum. During 'activity days' the curriculum was modified to promote 'togetherness' among children – cooperation, mutual support, flexibility – so that they could all engage in different subtasks constituting one common theme. Within such educational activities an outsider could not tell who was the support and who the mainstream teacher.

Teachers, however, also felt that they had to follow the requirements of the National Curriculum where the focus tended to be more on individualized subject-orientated tasks. In these circumstances collaboration among mainstream and support teachers was to be found mainly outside of the classroom at the level of planning. Collaborative activities were held by some teachers to be important in implementing the centralized curriculum reforms and in promoting integration.

It seemed that the nature and quality of teachers' working relationships influenced the way the requirements of the National Curriculum affected the education of children with special educational needs. As a mainstream teacher put it: 'It [the relationship] can make it or break it [integration]'. However, 'there is no such thing as "real" or "true" collaboration or collegiality. There are only different forms of collaboration and collegiality that have different consequences and serve different purposes' (Hargreaves 1994: 189).

Within the school particular forms of collaboration in different contexts were not without their problems and limitations. One informal form of collegiality was to be found usually in dinner times, when different support teachers working in the infants school gathered together on different days in a room other than the staffroom to discuss a variety of issues related to their work. This evolved out of some support teachers' feeling that working within an integrated resource could lead to a sense of 'being isolated'. This feeling was likely to have been reinforced by the lack of collaborative relationships across the whole school. It seemed that teachers were divided into separate groups belonging to the infants or the junior level, and to the mainstream or resource sector. The formation of the collaborative gathering among only infants support teachers indicated the subtle division of teachers into different and separate groups. As an infants support teacher put it:

> Another fear I have is that there is a sense of isolation when you are working in an integrated resource . . . Integrated resources to me seem to be many different things. They all seem to work in different ways. You've only got to look at the way colleagues work in the middle [junior] school and the way we [at the infants] work. We work from the same seat and yet we work in a very different way.

Collaborative activities between mainstream and support teachers were mutually agreed in meetings squeezed into breaks or any other circumstances where the teachers' presence in classrooms was not absolutely necessary (such as school assembly hours). Even though these activities were initiated by teachers they seemed to have acquired a structured, routinized and functional character. Teachers focused narrowly on planning together curricular activities and/or sharing ideas, in a way which appeared to contribute little to their existing expertise and understanding. Planning was mainly restricted to the specific and relatively short-term task of developing modified units of work for children with special educational needs. Often 'planning together' meant that the support teacher was following what the mainstream teacher had already planned:

> Jim, the teacher I always work with is good because he always produces things that he's going to do a couple of days before, so that I can make a modified version of it for the special needs children.

Collaborative activities remained at a functional level, which limited teachers' more critical reflection upon their practices and ideas in implementing the curricular reforms. In only one case did mainstream and support teachers work together not only outside of but within the class and enourage each other to reflect on their practices. This form of collaboration was based on a recognition that teachers can learn from each other by sharing and developing their expertise together. As the mainstream teacher put it:

It's [integration] a massive plus for me. It's a massive advantage for me because I've got another adult mind in the classroom that I can bounce ideas off and we can plan together and work together and sift out what's good and what's bad. It helps me to be a better teacher if there is another adult to criticize me when I need criticizing and to encourage me when I need encouraging and similarly the other way round. We're always telling each other 'You've made a mess of that' or 'You did that well, we'll do that again.' So to have another adult mind is a great thing.

The two teachers had blurred the boundaries of their roles as support and mainstream teachers by viewing themselves as two professionals who were responsible for the whole class. From participant observations it was noted that children with special educational needs were educated for the whole day within the ordinary class and withdrawal was kept to a minimum, taking place only when some children had to work individually with the speech therapist. As another teacher, referring to these two teachers, put it: 'Like R— and M— . . . they can have a completely different atmosphere in the classroom and because of that the situation of the two together is smoother.' Reversing the teacher's comment, it seemed that it was the nature and form of collegiality that the two teachers had developed which fostered the creation of a 'completely different classroom atmosphere'. This form of collegiality, promoting joint and critical work in classroom practice, seemed to be a key determinant in promoting inclusive educational activities. In the school as a whole, it was to be found mainly in the creation and implementation of 'activity days'. In the majority of other educational circumstances a strict division and separation of teachers' (mainstream and support) roles, priorities and responsibilities at the level of planning was based on a clear distinction of who was responsible for whom. This corresponded to teachers' perception of integration as a process of incorporating children who belonged to a different pedagogical category into ordinary classes. Some mainstream teachers claimed that it would have been more beneficial in academic terms if some children with special educational needs were educated in special schools. These teachers had absorbed the conflicting and confusing beliefs shaped by the old-fashioned and superficial 'integration versus segregation' argument. It was indicative that in the research interviews teachers focused highly on the social benefits of integration with little reference to its academic benefits. Behind this pattern, paradoxically, lies one of the reasons why teachers, despite controversial ideologies and practices, were in favour of promoting integrational practices in the way these were understood by them.

The role of the school in demystifying myths: perceptions and contradictions

All of the teachers who commented positively about integration saw major benefits for children's social education. Integration was perceived as a mechanism for promoting socialization between disabled and non-disabled children. Teachers claimed that integration broadened the life experiences of both mainstream and disabled children by raising awareness of the former on issues of disability and by educating them to tolerate and accept people who were different from them, and by providing the latter with role models from which they could learn appropriate social and other behavioural patterns. These aims were thought to be a major benefit of integration for children and for society in general; 'It was a lesson in life', as a teacher put it.

Often, when teachers were referring to the educational aspect of integration (i.e. content and delivery of the curriculum, and pace of work) and to classroom practices, they expressed the belief that disabled children would probably benefit more, academically, if they were in special schools. However, the majority of teachers resisted the idea of 'returning to segregated education' on the basis that the social advantages of integration outweighed the academic advantages of special provision (at special schools). Mousley *et al.* (1993: 66) found similar results in their exploration of teachers' attitudes towards integration: 'placing focus on the social . . . domain with little emphasis on academic possibilities is symptomatic of the beliefs teachers hold about disability; and reflects the typical curricula in segregated settings'. Teachers' responses showed that they rarely saw integration as an issue of equity; they tended to respond to it as an issue of 'moral sensitivity'.

As Quicke *et al.* have noted, moral sensitivity is a slippery concept. It can, however, be used to refer to the 'social feeling' that fosters motivation to engage in moral reasoning which is based mainly on the notion of concern for others. 'This basic feeling or sense is logically prior to rational decision-making and provides the moral setting for the teaching activity' (Quicke *et al.* 1990: 10). It was this element of moral sensitivity, different in nature and degree among different teachers, which inspired them to be positive towards the process of integration. The following positive responses derived from teachers' perception of the social benefits of integration:

I think it [integration] is all a bonus.

I think the advantages [of integration] for [all] the children far outweigh the disadvantages.

I think they [children with special educational needs] give us as much as they get.

I think it's a two-way process: that the children in the integrated resource do offer the school an awful lot. They receive an awful lot back, perhaps they receive more than they give; but they do give an awful lot to the school.

Integration was a 'good thing', a 'beneficial process', 'a way to go forward' on the basis that disabled children offered the opportunity for the other children to expand their social education and, in turn, disabled children were offered the opportunity (and sometimes the privilege) of mixing socially with their peers within an ordinary environment. Such an emphasis on only the social and moral benefits of integration, often influenced by a charitable type of humanism, seemed to hinder the translation of this moral commitment into the assertion of rights. It produced dilemmas for the teachers and often led to the perpetuation of myths, restricting even further the aims of integration. For instance, parents of disabled children were presented with the following restrictive choice:

> We say to parents when they come to look around, 'The setting is just to a certain extent a compromise. Do you want your child to read as quickly as possible [implying that this was the benefit of special schooling] or do you want them to learn to play with a group of children [implying that this was the benefit of integration]?'

Such restrictive 'choices' simplified the complex process of integration, created certain expectations at the expense of others and raised doubts about the responsibility of the school to educate *all* children. Understanding teachers' emphasis on the social and moral dimension of integration, often at the expense of inclusive pedagogical curricula, requires an exploration of their more general social experience (or lack of it) of disabled children/people.

All the teachers were asked whether or not they had any experience of people with Down's Syndrome outside the school community and/or prior to the establishment of the integrated resource at the school. The majority of the teachers referred to their childhood experience and their responses were indicative of the marginalization, isolation and social ostracism that people with Down's Syndrome had experienced in the past. The majority of the teachers had grown up in communities where children/people with Down's Syndrome seemed to be invisible. When they happened to be visible they were objects of 'fear of the unknown':

> I remember as a child being quite frightened by a Down's Syndrome lad who lived near me. He was older than I was. I can remember having that certain fear of this chap because he looked so different to me. I didn't know what he was capable of and I think people of our generation still have that fear.

Another teacher, as a child, had heard from her parents about 'this lady who had a Mongol child', while a third teacher had heard about how 'unfortunate' the sister of his mother's friend was in having a 'Mongol' child. The rest of the teachers claimed that they 'never came across them at all'. Children with Down's Syndrome were neither seen in the neighbourhood nor peers in ordinary schools. As a teacher put it in a mild way, the assumption was that 'Down's Syndrome children, in the past, tended to be children who weren't expected to be in mainstream education.' Throughout their early socialization process, teachers had grown up believing that ordinary schools were not for children with Down's Syndrome. The same teachers some years ago were called upon to achieve what previously had been strongly internalized as being unachievable: to educate children with Down's Syndrome. Thus it was no surprise that some teachers were hesitant and resisted the idea of including children with Down's Syndrome within ordinary academic classroom activities. Also, it was no surprise to listen to some teachers saying that initially they could not believe that they could actually teach these children to read and write or that they were surprised to find out that some of these children were 'actually quite bright'.

Many of the teachers, after interacting with the children with Down's Syndrome who were educated at the school, realized that most of the assumptions held by the general public (including themselves) were mainly based on prejudice. This prejudice had, according to teachers, developed out of the 'fear of the unknown' and had generated negative attitudes towards the children. The language that some of the teachers deployed in presenting these assumptions in regard to children with Down's Syndrome was indicative of the dominant language used by the general public when they themselves were children:

> They [children with Down's Syndrome] were thought of as being idiots, cretins, imbeciles with no abilities and no skills . . . I think a lot of ignorance surrounded these children.

> People with Down's Syndrome were thought to be dull, boisterous, large, you know, people thought that children with Down's Syndrome were monsters purely from their physical appearance, even though some of them are very nice to look at . . . Even today, I don't think that there are a lot of people who may appreciate that some people with Down's Syndrome can be very bright. I mean, different children [with Down's Syndrome] have different qualities, but they [people] perceive them as all Down's Syndrome, like you know, put all of them together: they are all Down's Syndrome, they are all noisy, they are all loud, they are not all that pleasant to look at.

> Well, I didn't have any experience [of children with Down's Syndrome] outside the school. I am certainly surprised at what they can do. I did not think they were capable of doing so much and I suspect a lot of people just dismiss them as not having much intelligence.

Through their own experience, some teachers learned that attitudinal responses towards disabled people were key determinants of their inclusion not only within education but within the wider community as well. The majority of teachers strongly believed that the process of integration was the best way to overcome such prejudices. They believed that the school can play a vital role in educating the general public in overcoming the 'fear of the unknown', when the general public is still young. Thus socializing and mixing with disabled people was held to be a great (if not the main) benefit of integration. It was the motivating force for changing attitudes and a moral stimulus for teachers to continue promoting integrational practices.

Why did teachers focus so much on the social aspect of integration, often to the expense of the quality of education that disabled children were receiving?

Why were teachers so strongly attached to the notion of normality and 'models of good social behaviour'? Perhaps we should bear in mind Uditsky's suggestion:

> Exclusion and segregation were built on centuries of devaluation. Those of us who are parents and teachers have not grown up or been immersed in a culture where inclusion and friendship with persons with a disability is an ordinary and typical life occurrence.
>
> (Uditsky 1993: 90)

Conclusion

So far I have attempted to locate the question of inclusive education within the wider educational context. The exploration and understanding of teachers' attitudes towards the integration process was grounded in the educational context within which these attitudes have developed. In this way, the analysis was geared towards the exploration of these institutionalized educational processes which seemed to influence and shape teachers' attitudes towards integration, and to provide a basis for retaining the distinctions between 'normal' and 'special' – or in this case, 'resource children'.

Teachers' attitudes towards the integration process tended to be conflicting and often confusing because the notion of integration did not have a single definition. Its meaning was rather to be found in the context and purpose of its use, depending on several educational (im)practicalities. In practice teachers' willingness and commitment in promoting integrational practices were highly influenced by the conditions within which they had to work; these conditions tended to make the commitment to inclusive education more difficult to maintain.

It has been emphasized that the degree of teachers' satisfaction in their work was under threat. Teachers were concerned and anxious about the conflicting demands they were expected to fulfil. On the one hand, they wanted to spend time with the children and approach their work conscientiously and caringly. On the other, they had to deal with the sheer volume of the government's sweeping changes in educational legislation. Teachers were under intense pressure to accomplish what they were expected to, even though some of the legislative requirements (such as bureaucratic and administrative ones) were considered as 'a waste of valuable teaching time'.

Teachers also found their established views of 'good practice' in conflict with the government's commercially-driven values. Commitment to the importance of integration was often seen as an additional burden because it was in conflict with the pressure to 'improve results'; and the intensification of competition was contrary to the teachers' educational principles.

Furthermore, it was noted that teachers' perceptions about 'resource children' were influenced by several complex institutionalized processes. These processes often led teachers to focus on within-the-child difficulties in justifying not only their attitudes towards integration but also the quality and the nature of the education provided. Children with special educational needs were in danger of experiencing a higher degree of exclusion within ordinary classrooms because of the intensification and mechanization of the teaching activity, which reinforced a restrictive notion of learning and a specific image of children as absorbers of enormous amounts of information. Also teachers had to struggle to avoid 'fitting the children to the needs of the curriculum' – there was an increasing tendency to reformulate children's needs so as to respond to the demands of a market-led educational system. These difficulties were compounded by the fiscal crisis, which made it nearly impossible for the school to have sufficient resources to meet all of the expected goals.

However, despite the above contradictions and complexities, the majority of teachers were positive in promoting integrational practices. All teachers who commented positively about integration saw major benefits for children's social education. Their positive attitudes originated from a recognition that integration was the best way of overcoming prejudice. This recognition was based on their experience of growing up in communities where disabled children (e.g. children with Down's Syndrome) were either invisible or were targets of curiosity, pity and fear. They felt a moral responsibility to contribute to a positive generational change, to a more caring culture. Often, however, teachers' moral sensitivity was influenced by a charitable type of humanism at the expense of other educational/pedagogical benefits that could derive from the integration process. Thus integration was strongly presented as a mechanism for educating mainstream children to tolerate and accept people who are different than themselves.

All the teachers placed a great emphasis on the social aspect of integration because they believed that peers' attitudes towards disabled children were key determinants of their inclusion. Indeed, such attitudes have been identified as a crucial social parameter influencing the nature and quality of integration within ordinary educational communities. In a lot of social contexts disabled children do seem to 'suffer' a measure of 'social ostracism' (Thomas 1982: 3) and social isolation by their peers. By exploring peers' attitudes, we explore the social infrastructure of the school and the messages children receive from their environment regarding issues of disability. It further sheds light on the complex process of how children/people make sense of their relationships and friendships with their disabled and non-disabled peers. In other words, it helps us to identify the degree of complexity of the social barriers to be overcome in the development of a more inclusive understanding for communities. The following chapters consequently focus on children's perspectives toward the notion of integration and the way(s) they construct their socio-interactional realities with their peers (both disabled and non-disabled). This includes the relationships and tensions between themselves and the reality of their everyday socio-educational lives.

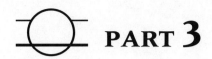 **PART 3**

CHILDREN'S PERSPECTIVES

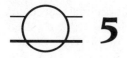 **5**

Integration: the children's point of view

A photograph portraying two girls – Claire, who was non-disabled, and Sam, with Down's Syndrome – acted as the stimulus for initiating discussions with the children at the school on the integration process and the formation of interpersonal relationships between disabled and non-disabled individuals (See Appendix 3). None of the children had met Claire or Sam. The children had a first-hand experience of being educated 'with' – at least alongside – peers with Down's Syndrome and thus their accounts were both responses to fictional/hypothetical questions and reflections of their actual everyday schooling experience. The transition from the fictional/hypothetical world to their own real world took place in a 'natural' way. The picture generated questions and created 'realities' drawn from an already existing ideological and cultural environment – that of the childrens' own experience (see Vlachou 1995b).

In the initial phase of describing Claire and Sam and creating a story about them, almost all of the 103 children indicated that Sam was younger than Claire. This reflects the tendency of 'ordinary' children to perceive disabled children as being younger than their actual chronological age (see Strain 1984; Lewis and Lewis 1988). However, to be 'younger', in the way children used that term within this specific context, also meant being 'less mature' and 'less clever'. Age was considered as a reason for the two girls not attending the same class.

Only a small number of pupils thought that both Claire and Sam were attending the same class, indicating that the hypothetical class consisted of mixed-aged students, similar to the ones they themselves were attending:

Pupil A: They're going to the same class/
Pupil B: Yeah, 'cos, like, in classes they have 9- and 10-year-olds or 8 and 9.

Pursuing the discussion further, however, it was revealed that reasons other than age affected children's judgements regarding the educational placement of the two girls. The first questions that the photograph raised for children were related to issues concerning the perceived identity of the two girls, and this seemed to influence their subsequent responses significantly. Thus children were initially engaged in placing Claire and Sam into certain social categories: 'normal' and 'disabled'. These categories were used as the basis for drawing inferences about the girls even though they knew nothing about them beyond their preconceptions of the characteristics of each category. The children used these assumptions to explain the girls' perceived behaviour, to make predictions about them and to form perceptions of their place in the general social order.

The first issue to emerge in the process of creating the identity of Sam was related to the wider social effort of promoting the idea of a continuum of 'handicap'. Please note that the identity of 'Pupil A' and so on will normally be different in each transcription.

> *Interviewer*: They're not in the same class?
> *Pupil A*: No, because Sam looks different than Claire.
> *Interviewer*: What's the difference?
> *Pupil A*: Her teeth.
> *Interviewer*: Is her teeth a reason to be in a different class?
> *Pupil B*: No, but she's [Sam] not exactly the same as Claire. She looks like ... She's a bit like, like Spyros [a peer with Down's Syndrome] and Patricia/
> *Pupil C*: or Nick [a peer identified as a 'resource student'] and Kathy [ditto].
> *Pupil A*: Kathy is 10 but she's in Mrs B—'s group but she's coping in the proper class.
> *Interviewer*: I think I've lost you. You said that Sam looks like Spyros and Patricia/
> *Pupil A*: 'cos she doesn't look like she knows everything, like spelling things.
> *Pupil C*: Like Patricia ... [pause] ... Like Patricia, she doesn't know much and she [Sam] looks like she doesn't know much.
> *Pupil B*: She looks like Kathy/
> *Pupil A*: Kathy knows some things and others she doesn't, but Patricia doesn't know anything like that.

From participant observations in the class attended by the above group of pupils and in discussions with both the mainstream and support teachers it was noted that the four children mentioned above (Kathy, Spyros, Patricia and Nick) were identified as resource pupils. Spyros was a pupil with Down's Syndrome, Patricia was identified by the teachers as a child with autistic tendencies, while Kathy and Nick were identified as children with learning difficulties. The above account indicates children's struggle to place Sam into a category which accorded with her perceived degree of 'handicap' or 'individual needs'.

It seems that the idea of a continuum of 'handicap' engenders conflict when thinking about disability and disabled people, by acknowledging that different disabled people or, in this case, 'resource children' exhibit different strengths and weaknesses. But the philosophy of a continuum of 'needs' or 'handicap' did not necessarily alleviate the barrier between 'normal' and 'disabled'. As Quicke has already suggested,

> One could argue that the notion of a continuum of handicap reinforces rather than punctures stereotypes because the barrier between 'normal' and 'handicapped' is retained in this idea. Persons may be categorized as mildly, severely or profoundly handicapped but they still have a handicapped identity.
>
> (Quicke *et al.* 1990: 121)

In the pupils' words:

> *Pupil A* :　She [Sam] is like Peter [a peer with Down's Syndrome] . . . Nick and Philip I don't think *they're so brain damaged* like not so much as Peter [emphasis added].

> *Pupil A*:　She's like Kris. Kris is handicapped. Is Kris handicapped?
> *Pupil B*:　I don't know. *He's not as handicapped as Peter* but he's a resource student. I know that [emphasis added].

All children with Down's Syndrome were classified by their peers as being 'very handicapped', which meant they were 'more handicapped' than their 'handicapped' peers – with all the social connotations that implied. The struggle to categorize according to a continuum of 'handicap' centred mainly on the rest of the so-called 'resource' pupils, for whom the epithet 'handicapped' was still retained by the majority of children, depending on the perceived degree, severity and intensity of the 'handicap'.

The implicit idea behind the making of comparisons was that at one end of the continuum were the 'normal' children, and at the other end the disabled children; the assumption was that the 'normal' are always better than the disabled pupils, who were comparatively 'always slow' and 'needed help'. Even in cases where children could identify ordinary pupils in their own classes as 'being slow' or having difficulties in learning, the differentiation between 'normal' and 'disabled' still remained on the basis of a perceived quantifiable degree of difficulty (i.e. 'always' slow):

> *Pupil A*:　Sam needs more help than Claire/
> *Pupil B*:　She needs a special teacher 'cos she's backwards.
> *Interviewer*:　Backwards? What does backwards mean?
> *Pupil A*:　She's slow. Like Norma Philips [an ordinary classmate] . . . She's on the last question and she had about 20 attempts at it and got them all wrong/
> *Interviewer*:　So Norma is 'backwards'?
> *Pupil C*:　No. She [Norma] is not backwards. She can do it but she gets everything wrong . . . Sam is like Nina [a peer with Down's Syndrome].
> *Pupil B*:　Oh yeah. She's always slow.

In comparing academic achievement, children seemed to focus on the abilities of ordinary pupils and the weaknesses of the disabled pupils, magnifying in this way the differences between 'normal' and disabled children. Even though they were aware that ordinary pupils have difficulties and needs as well, often, in creating Claire's identity, they seemed to have a particular image of 'the ideal ordinary pupil' not very different from the one reinforced by the new educational trends or those desired by a large proportion of teachers:

> *Pupil A*: She [Claire] does very good work. She likes maths, science, art, English and colouring . . . She doesn't need much help 'cos she's clever/
> *Pupil B*: She can do anything.

Describing Claire:

> *Pupil A*: She's good at everything. She's good at maths, at English, at Sports . . .

> *Pupil A*: She's clever, hard working, fast/
> *Pupil B*: Intelligent/
> *Pupil A*: She's like Susan Smith [an ordinary peer]. She knows everything.

Juxtaposed to Claire's perceived academic abilities were Sam's perceived 'inabilities':

> *Pupil A*: She's not able to write like other people can.

> *Pupil B*: She doesn't know as many words as ordinary people.

> *Pupil C*: She's not able to write very well [and] she might be a bit deaf.

> *Pupil D*: She's not good at colouring, she's scribbling and she works in a rush.

> *Pupil E*: She doesn't know how to spell, how to draw and things like that.

> *Pupil F*: She's slow, I don't think she's as good as Claire. She needs more help than Claire 'cos she makes quite a lot of mistakes.

> *Pupil G*: She's rubbish, she cannot do English, she cannot do gymnastics. She's rubbish . . . when she's writing she's always scribbling, she's too heavy and she goes like that [imitating].

Within this well-established ideological process and in accordance with the dominant identified pattern, it was only Sam who needed help and the dilemma was whether Sam could benefit from attending an ordinary school and in what way. The already existing alternative to the ordinary school was the special school, and thus the integration–segregation debate surfaced with almost no prompting from the interviewer:

> *Pupil A*: I think that Claire goes to a school like ours and Sam to a special school.

Interviewer: Why?

Pupil A: If you send Claire to the same school as Sam then it would be a waste of money 'cos only Sam needs the help and Claire's all right. She can do good work like us in our class.

However, the issue was much more complicated than the above account indicates, since the same pupil elsewhere during the discussion offered a number of reasons for justifying his opinion that it would be better for Sam to be educated in an ordinary school. Conflicts and contradictions were prevalent in children's responses. In trying to make sense of these tensions and conflicts I was helped by Quicke *et al.*'s (1991) critique of the 'universality of prejudice' thesis and its connection with education. A central point of Quicke *et al.*'s position is the significance of the argumentative aspect of life. As they maintain:

> Living within a tradition can often be a contradictory experience and our 'common sense' contains contrary elements which are widespread throughout the culture. Thus we are not only aware of points 'for and against', but often ourselves use contradictory arguments on different occasions.
>
> (Quicke 1991: 51)

Unresolved tensions

From the vast majority of Year 4, 5 and 6 pupils it was felt that Sam should be educated in an ordinary school, identifying the ordinary school with their own – 'in a school like ours'. Pupils' justifications differed. As the following accounts indicate, some children thought it 'natural' that Sam should attend an ordinary school, just as their disabled peers were doing:

Pupil A: She [Sam] goes to a normal school, 'cos Helen and Spyros go to an ordinary school/

Pupil B: Yeah, because Peter and Spyros go to a normal school so she can go to a normal school.

Pupil A: She [Sam] goes to a normal school. Like Peter, Caroline, Philip and George are in our school.

Pupil B: I think Sam should be able to come here [to their school] and sit next to Mrs B— [a support teacher].

Pupil A: Well, Sam can come to this school 'cos we have handicapped people in our class anyway.

In other cases, some children thought that Sam should attend an ordinary school as a matter of personal preference. The children were quite clear and concise in their responses, assuming that Sam's friends were attending an ordinary school or that Sam was already attending an ordinary school and thus she had already established some friendships. Other pupils supported the idea of integration by enumerating what they thought as being the 'main problems' of attending a special school. One of these problems, expressed mainly by Year 4 and 5 pupils, was associated with the perception that special schools are boarding schools and thus expensive.

The second 'main' problem of attending a special school was associated with distance. Some children thought that disabled pupils should be able to be educated at the school nearest to them. This presumed that special schools were somewhere far away. In their confusion children often indicated that their own school was the nearest for disabled children, probably having in mind only one of their disabled peers, who happened to be a local resident as well. In so thinking they failed to take account of the so-called 'resource pupils' who came to school by taxi or minibus from other, distant areas.

However, it was not unusual to hear children wondering: 'Disabled children can come to this school? We aren't handicapped are we?' or 'We are not a special school. We are a normal school.' Although such a response ostensibly addresses the placement of a disabled individual, in practice its concern focuses on questions of identification and categorization often related to the complex process of classifying self by classifying others. Some children, in clarifying that they were different from their disabled peers, indicated that the latter were not doing the same work as them, 'the normals'.

Also children's tendency to focus on the within-the-child difficulties, by emphasizing disabled peers' inabilities to achieve academically, led them to the assumption that integration is a process that presupposes certain conditions:

Pupil A: Because they [disabled pupils] don't have the same ability like me, like doing maths or English or going around the school but these children, the ones that haven't got the same ability as us, they need separate classes, like Peter.

Pupil B: They need a special teacher and special work 'cos if they have the work that we do they never get it done.

In some cases the educational plan that children offered was specific and not very different from either the one many teachers, and particularly psychologists, espouse for the educational placement of disabled children, or some variation of the plan already in existence:

Pupil A: She [Sam should go to] a special [school] first and then go on to, like, a school like ours/

Pupil B: When, like, you're downstairs [at infants school] she might have gone into a special one and she might have gone downstairs to a special classroom but when she's upstairs [junior school] she goes in, like, just a normal class.

Pupil A: She'll be like Helen . . . They'll see how clever she was and then they'd know which class to put her in and do all the arrangements.

The arrangements seemed to be quite specific. Children, in projecting the discursive practices within which they have learned to think about the process of integration and in adopting the main arguments deployed by adults in defining the notion of integration, thought that it would be beneficial for Sam (who represented disabled children) to attend an ordinary school, provided that:

Pupil A: They have special teachers to look after them.

Pupil B: They have special things to help them.

Pupil C: She [Sam] should have her own personal class because she's not as good as her friend [Claire]. She needs to have like special care treatment.

Pupil D: they have teachers who can do special work. They have special classrooms.

Pupil E: They've got special equipment and some special teachers that could help them to understand things and special computers so that they know what they're doing . . . With the special equipment it will be easier for Sam to understand.

Even though resources are necessary for creating a more inclusive education, the term 'special' seemed to be such a dominant feature in children's responses that it was often one of the main reasons used in justifying the exclusion of disabled children from ordinary schools:

Pupil A: It's better to go to a special school because she'll have more special teachers, like Mr H— or Mrs S— [support teachers] who look after, like, backwards people to make 'em go forward . . . They [special teachers] can help them [disabled people] better there [at a special school]. They can help them to walk better and talk. They help them to write properly.

Pupil B: They've [at a special school] got more special teachers like Mrs M— and Mr S— [support teachers] who'll spend time with them [disabled children] rather than the other children.

Pupil C: It's better [for Sam] to go to a special school because she might not get much attention here.

Pupil D: There's more stuff she can do [at a special school] and things they can help her with. There's more special equipment.

It was interesting that while the majority of children indicated that special schools were better for disabled children because they had special staff, almost no one indicated that their school lacked the above prerequisite. The justification for segregated education was based not on getting attention or having special teachers, but on having more special teachers and on getting more attention.

In understanding children's accounts it would be a mistake to ignore that such responses are probably based on a realistic appraisal of the educational structures that children themselves experience. Children's accounts may indeed reflect their true concern for the education of disabled children. The fact that at overcrowded ordinary schools children are perceived as one of the crowd should not be underestimated. For instance, it was shown in the ORACLE study of junior school classrooms that children interacted with their teachers for only 2.3 per cent of the time as individuals and only 15.8 per cent of the time as a member of a group or the whole class (Galton *et al.* 1980 as cited in Pollard 1992). As Pollard indicates, 'these are dramatically small over-all figures, but ones which are perhaps inevitable given the teacher–pupil ratios which are deemed to be acceptable in primary school classrooms' (p. 41). Children, perceiving disabled pupils as needing more help than themselves and judging from their own experience of how difficult it is for teachers to spend a sufficient amount of time in responding to individual needs, could have been led to the assumption that it would be better for their disabled peers to be educated in a special environment where more attention would be offered to them. In fact, from participant observations in three classes it was noted that 'resource pupils' were often overlooked in busy classrooms, even in cases were activities were designed ostensibly to include all students. Under the present circumstances (see Chapter 3) and in view of the established differentiation of 'normal' and disabled groups of children, it was not coincidental that some pupils, expressing their own concerns as well as reflecting teachers' opinions, went even further by claiming that special teachers were necessary because otherwise:

Pupil A: Mr R— [the mainstream teacher] would have to help all the children and the handicapped children as well.
Pupil B: It wouldn't be fair for Mr W— [mainstream teacher] 'cos he's got two kinds of children ['normal' and disabled] and he'd spend more time on disabled than he would on us so he'll have to rely on us to behave.
Pupil C: If Mr R— [mainstream teacher] were just teaching all of the class, he couldn't because they're, like, two people to handle at once: there's the whole class and there's the disabled part of the class.

While statements such as the second one above express children's concern for their own educational experience as well, the responses as a whole did not differ from those offered by mainstream teachers who, under the current pressures, viewed as their first priority the education of 'ordinary' children, leaving to support/'special' teachers the education of disabled students.

However, it is one thing to say that children require more contact time with their teachers and another to specify that it is only disabled children who are in need of individual attention by special teachers. An emphasis on being 'special' constitutes the discursive practice through which children come to view the notion of integration. If we consider that such an emphasis maintains the process of labelling by perpetuating the 'ordinary' – 'special' dualism, then children need to view disabled people as not being different from themselves, while at the same time they must learn to think and act within a linguistic system in which such distinctions are deeply rooted. Disabled children were considered to need 'special' teachers, who in turn were often perceived as acquiring some particular characteristics that made them special. For instance, 'special' teachers were seen as necessary for the education of 'special children', not only because of their functional role ('they know what they're doing with handicapped people') but also because of the characteristics attributed to someone who is involved with the education of disabled children. 'Special' teachers were often thought to be 'very nice, and kind and patient and so another teacher might not have been as patient':

> *Pupil A*: Like Mrs H— is prepared to take them [disabled peers] aside and she's prepared to work with them in different things and she doesn't get impatient if she gives them something to do and they're not doing it, she is not saying 'Oh, I am going to teach normal people.' She actually takes the time and patience to teach these children.

Such images imply that limitless patience and kindness are necessary characteristics of those involved with disabled children. In this way the importance of 'special' teachers was strengthened even further by children.

At the same time, however, and in addition to the notion of being 'special', which implies that problems are located within the child, many pupils were aware that the process of integration could be problematic because of difficulties imposed by the school environment. Expressing a limited perception of the concept 'environment', they identified two areas which seemed to be of great importance in influencing their opinions regarding the integration of disabled peers: the structure of the building and ordinary pupils' behaviour towards disabled peers. Both areas were sources of controversy.

As far as the building was concerned, children focused on the architectural obstacles that their school would impose on children with physical disabilities:

> *Pupil A*: They've not done it very good because what if they're in wheelchairs with all these stairs. They should have this, like, I've forgotten what they call it, but it's like a ramp going downstairs.

Most of Year 6 pupils, drawing from their past experience, offered a number of examples of physically disabled pupils who had to leave their school because of difficulty using the stairs:

> *Pupil A*: There was a girl called Fay and she was in our class. She had to be in a wheelchair and then she left school and went to another one because when it was time for her to go upstairs, there were too many stairs for her and she would have had problems . . . They don't have any slopes.
>
> *Pupil B*: Mike Thomas used to be here, but he had to leave from the school because he was using a wheelchair and he couldn't come up. There aren't any lifts.

Pupil C: We had a girl that left because she was in a wheelchair and she couldn't come up. I think they're supposed to have lifts.

Pupil D: When we were downstairs there was somebody in a wheelchair and we were going to have, like, a lift but they thought it was too much so she had to go to another school.

The existence of stairs was used by some children as a reason for justifying their opinion that Sam could not be educated at their school. On this basis, many of them chose Claire when asked who they would have liked to come to their school, even though there were no indications in the picture that Sam was a physically disabled individual or had any difficulties with walking:

Pupil A: I wouldn't bring Sam [to school] because if she's handicapped or something and she's in a wheelchair then it'd be hard for her to get around in our school 'cos at playtime you have to go down some stairs.
Interviewer: Is she sitting in a wheelchair?
Pupil B: She's just sitting in a normal chair. She might have a wheelchair somewhere else in the house.

While children indicated an awareness of the difficulties that physically disabled children would encounter in an environment that had not been designed for them, practical difficulties were often used as a rationalization of exclusion. This found reinforcement in combination with another area of controversy related to the social relations between ordinary and disabled children.

The vast majority of children expressed the opinion that it would have been beneficial for Sam and for disabled people to be educated in an ordinary school because in this way they would have the opportunity to mix with ordinary children:

Pupil A: She'll mix in. She can play with other people.

Pupil B: She'll mix with normal people.

Pupil C: Ordinary schools are better so that they can make friends with other people.

Pupil D: [In an ordinary school] they've got lots of friends to rely on and to play with in the playground. Like Peter, he's enjoying being in the class because he's not surrounded by all handicapped people. He's surrounded by other persons like me and Pauline.

Pupil E: She [Sam] could have some good friends, be cared about and . . . [unclear] her friends will make her join in. She might not get bullied.

Pupil F: She [Sam] can go to an ordinary school, 'cos she will mix with normal people like us and she can learn more. Like she could do songs, she can learn how to play properly and do things like normal people do, so that she doesn't have to be relying on people all the time.

As Quicke *et al.* (1990: 117) indicate, 'recognition of the value of mixing is regarded as a progressive development'. For the pupils of this study, mixing with other people, with 'the normals', was important not only in making friends but in being perceived as normal:

Pupil A: They'll treat them as normal – they won't cast them aside.

Pupil B: He [a peer with Down's Syndrome] has lots and lots of friends. He wouldn't know that he has all these friends because he goes around and says hello to everybody and the others just treat him like a normal person.

Pupil C: I know what he's [a peer with Down's Syndrome] enjoying. He's enjoying it when we treat him as a normal person.

Pupil D: [In an ordinary school] she'll have friends and she'll be taught by teachers as a normal person.

Pupil E: She might have [in an ordinary school] more friends and more people to help her because she'll be getting to the standards – to what other people are now.

To be perceived of as a normal person was of great significance, especially to older pupils. As was the case with teachers, children indicated a strong association between the process of integration and the process of acquiring 'normalcy'. Being perceived as normal and/or being treated as normal was regarded by the children as a productive learning experience for their disabled peers. However, being 'normal' meant 'being like us'; conflict originated from the fundamental ideology expressed by the majority of pupils that 'disabled people are not like us'. 'Treating' disabled people as 'normal' while at the same time perceiving the normality of their social identity as fragile and negotiable seemed to be an inherent contradiction, creating not only conflicts in perceptions and actions but a particular notion of humanism as well. While 'mixing with "normal" children' seemed to be a justification for integration, it also constituted an area for justifying exclusion on the grounds that these children needed to be protected from their 'normal' peers because they would be picked on by them:

Pupil A: It is better for Sam to go to a private [special] school where she can mix with people of her own kind . . . If you're at a special school most people are like you.

Pupil B: It's better [for Sam] to go to a special school because at a special school everyone's like that and they can't make fun of her. They're all like that really . . . they are the same and they cannot torment each other.

Pupil C: [It's better for disabled children to go to special schools] because all the other people are handicapped and there are not going to be other people to pick on them.

Such accounts reveal that disabled children were indeed perceived by other children as being different than themselves, and that this difference was a potential source of being (to use the children's term) 'tormented'. Moreover, the reasoning behind such responses was strongly based on the assumption/stereotype that all disabled children are the same and thus one could not 'torment' the other. The word 'torment' was used as a synonym to 'calling names', 'teasing', 'making fun of' or 'pulling faces'. Simultaneously, however, children were aware that the problem lay not only in the 'differences' exhibited by disabled children but also in the behaviour of the 'non-disabled' children towards disabled individuals.

'Picking-on' behaviour was clearly significant because, as the children's accounts suggested, it ranked in importance with ideas of being 'special' and special equipment as a reason for considering integration as a problem. Surprisingly, while children saw 'picking-on' behaviour as a main problem of the disabled child (Sam) attending an ordinary school, they no longer saw teasing disabled students as such a great problem when referring to their own disabled peers.

The study findings relating to the formation of interpersonal relations suggested that 'picking on disabled children' was a far more complicated phenomenon than it seemed to be at first glance – it was part of or even a consequence of a much wider social process. The issue of picking on and being picked on by someone else can be understood only within the wider context of the children's struggle to establish and position the 'self' and the 'other' within childhood culture. These struggles were enacted in the realm of power relationships surrounding one of the most common themes in children's culture, that of competence. Every child had experienced, to a different extent and in different ways, the sorts of power games associated with the formation of relationships (see Davies 1982). These power games in turn influenced and were influenced by the image and the status of each child within group situations. In other words, every child had experienced 'picking-on behaviour'. As a pupil put it, 'Everyone gets picked on every once in a while.'

'Picking-on' behaviour was part of the power games included in forming relationships; it was probably what lay behind the actual action of 'picking on someone' that was more important than the behaviour itself. For instance, pupils were aware that terms such as 'spaz', 'thick' and often 'handicapped' were 'rotten' and/or 'awful' names to call someone. However, they continued to use them when referring to some of their peers who were by no means all 'resource pupils', although such pupils were included as well. It was not the label itself that was 'awful' but the aims of using such labels. As Edgerton (1967: 145) has noted, such labels 'not only serve as a humiliating, frustrating, and discrediting stigma in the conduct of one's life in the community, [they] also serve to lower one's self esteem to such a nadir of worthlessness that the life of a person so labelled is scarcely worth living'. Translating this into the children's reality, picking on peers by using such derogatory names was a way of lowering the other's status and self-esteem, a way of asserting superiority or indicating rejection by a particular group at a particular time.

The overwhelming majority of pupils probably mentioned 'picking-on' behaviour as a negative aspect of integrating disabled pupils because 'picking-on' behaviour was an integral element within childhood culture; the ones who were at the receiving end of such behaviour were those who had lower status within that culture.

In the youngest class of pupils who participated in this study (Years 1 and 2), most of the boys indicated a group of four girls, known as 'the brainy ones', as people who picked on everybody. They were thus viewed as a potential source of difficulty for disabled pupils. At the same time, however, the vast majority of the girls of this class named three boys, 'the naughty ones', as those involved in aggressive behaviour, though not necessarily towards their disabled peers.

In older classes, very few students of either gender thought it would be mainly boys who were going to pick on Sam. Others, both boys and girls, drawing from their own experience thought that it would be the Year 7s, and of these mainly the boys who played football at a specific playground, who were going to pick on Sam:

> *Interviewer*: Who do you think is going to pick on Sam?
> *Pupil A*: No one in our class, somebody from another class.
> *Pupil B*: Like Year 7.
> *Interviewer*: Year 7?
> *Pupil A*: Yeah, 'cos she's younger and she just started/

> Like Year 7s, they're really rough. They bully a lot because like, you're younger than them and, like, you're smaller than them and they think you can't do as much things as them because they're older.

Younger pupils, both girls and boys, as well as older boys perceived as 'weak', seemed to base their statements on their own experience with the older and 'tougher' male pupils who expressed their superiority and macho identity by forming exclusive football teams. Most of these boys, however, viewed their actions as 'part of the fun' by including disabled peers, mainly boys, in their teams. From participant observations it was noted that while children with Down's Syndrome were often not included in these teams because, according to the 'leaders' of the team, 'they can't understand the rules of the game', a physically disabled peer, in contrast, was 'one of the lads' in the football team. Most of the boys did not view themselves as oppressing their disabled peers even though they indicated that the girls were more likely to become friends with Sam and be more caring towards her. It is difficult, however, to distinguish whether this response was offered because Sam was a disabled individual or because she was female.

The children's accounts did not reveal the gender issue in children's attitudes towards integration as much as expected. Quicke's (1989) analysis on disability and gender relations can shed some light on this issue. According to the findings of his study,

> The girls' generalisations from their own experiences of boys' assertive

behaviour were particularly understandable, but this, plus their own emerging allegiance to traditional female images led to their misrecognising the boys' potential for making positive relationships with mentally handicapped [*sic*] pupils. Similarly, boys could have been helped to a realisation of the inconsistencies and ambiguities in their own position: like, for instance, the contradiction between their emphasis on *equality* and *dignity* in relation to mentally handicapped [*sic*] and their emergent sexist attitudes in relation to girls.

(Quicke 1989: 142, emphasis in original)

An affective aspect of integration

Children's responses to the question of whether they liked being in the same class as disabled peers revealed some interesting findings. Year 1 and 2 pupils were negative about the idea of being educated together with the so-called 'resource' children. The reasoning used to justify such feelings was based more on children's perceived images of their peers rather than the process of integration itself. In their responses children focused mainly on their 'resource' peers' behaviour, with greater emphasis on the behaviour of their female peer with Down's Syndrome rather than the behaviour of the rest of their 'resource' peers (i.e. she is naughty, she hides my things, she kicks me, she's nipping me).

Older pupils claimed that they liked being in the same class as their disabled peers. As one pupil put it, 'it makes it different', even though the notion of 'different' had a variety of meanings and reasonings. Pupils liked to be educated with disabled peers because they perceived it as a beneficial experience for themselves. They were 'learning' out of this experience even though the type of learning had multiple dimensions. Some claimed that it was beneficial seeing that disabled children were able to do things as well:

> *Pupil A*: It's good to see that people like Kelly and Spyros can do things, like Kelly and Spyros are handicapped people and it's good when they're dancing with us and when we do PE together.

> *Pupil B*: I like it 'cos if you can see some handicapped people doing some good colouring you think 'God, I can't do as good colouring as that' and today Peter did some good colouring and everybody started looking at it and going 'Oh' 'cos it was really good.

> *Pupil C*: I like having them in the class. Sometimes they show us things that disabled people can do. Like, if someone is in a wheelchair he shows you how they use them and things like that, how you steer them.

Others claimed that they liked to be with disabled pupils because they learned 'how to cope with them'. As the following accounts indicate, the language used is not very different from that some adults employ when referring to the benefits of integration for non-disabled pupils:

Pupil A: You learn to cope with those. Like if you want to be a teacher you learn to cope with those when you're young and then when you get older you know what to, like, do when they're doing something.

Pupil B: You learn how to cope with them and then when you're somewhere public and there's a disabled person there and he or she needs help, you know how to cope with them.

Some pupils liked the fact that

Pupil C: Sometimes they [disabled peers] get the same work like us and if they cannot understand then we do it again and we understand it better.

However, according to the dominant pattern, children enjoyed having disabled peers in the same class for two basic reasons: first, 'it was more fun', and second, they could help them. 'It was more fun' to have disabled peers in the class either because

Pupil A: You get more people in the class and there's more fun when there's more people inside. Like I like Mrs B— and Mrs S— [the support teachers] and today I was messing with Helen [a peer identified as a 'resource' student] and Mrs B— was telling us to be quiet and then Mrs S— walked in and said 'Yeah, shut up' and I thought that was funny and everybody [including the teachers] started laughing.

or because

Pupil B: I like Spyros [a student with Down's Syndrome] to be in my class because he's funny and he's a non-stop joker.

Pupil C: I like it because they make us laugh. Like Patricia when she says 'Hello Mr R—' and she makes us laugh and we like Mr R— when he tells us jokes.

Characterizations such as 'being funny' and 'making jokes' were perceived by the majority of students as positive personality traits. Furthermore, from participant observations it was noted that children either welcomed or purposely created 'funny' situations so as to break the formalities, the tensions, the stress and/or the boredom of the classroom environment. However, it was difficult to distinguish whether they were laughing with or at their particular disabled peer, who happened to do or say something that was perceived as 'funny'. In other words, it was difficult to understand whether it was the 'deviation' of the act that generated laughter or whether children concentrated more on the social interaction and the sharing of the social situation.

Children liked being in the same class with disabled pupils because they had the opportunity to help them. While the notion of 'help' is a desirable social feature among people, it can have different underlying connotations, especially when it is strongly linked with a humanism based on needs (and its correlation, 'the needy') rather than rights within a society dominated by notions of competence, individualism and the ability to be self-sufficient. As Thomas indicates,

> We know that our society is in part based on an ethic which gives emphasis to self-sufficiency and independence, status and success, power, and wealth; and while it acknowledges that there are disadvantaged individuals and groups whose needs can legitimately be met, there is a survival of belief in self-sufficiency such as to make the recipient of public and private assistance feel subordinate and inferior.
>
> (Thomas 1982: 72)

Quicke's study of interventions in pupil–pupil interactions, like those of peer tutoring schemes and special educational needs, sheds further light on this point. According to his findings, situations within which one person provides help and the other receives it 'are not as straightforwardly a "good" thing as many of their protagonists may imagine. Far from being a positive intervention in the pupils' world they may paradoxically highlight and reinforce the negative aspects of pupil culture to the detriment of special needs [*sic*] pupils'(Quicke 1986: 163). That is because any such interventions should be grounded on a thorough understanding of pupils' meanings and the social processes which generate them. According to this study, children thought of their disabled peers as 'always needing help' because of their 'inabilities', and thus they were perceived not as people who are helped but as 'helped people' – a status which places dependency over personality. Such a status had negative consequences for disabled children; they were perceived as having a passive role in situations where they were being helped by their non-disabled peers. Consequently many children claimed that ordinary children often 'got fed up' with helping disabled children and this was offered as a possible reason why 'normal' children didn't like to be with disabled children.

Nevertheless, it was heartening to hear that many children liked being educated with their disabled peers. Those who expressed negative feelings claimed that they did not like the 'disruption' caused by the existence of disabled peers in their class:

Pupil A: I like it [being in the same class with Spyros] because he does jokes and we laugh, but sometimes what I don't like is when you're telling him to be quiet and you are trying to say to him to be quiet and the teacher is asking you to write something, you have missed it and you get done.

Pupil B: They don't let me go on with my work, 'cos Nina will hide all the rubbers and she disrupts us and we have to start our work from the beginning.

Pupil C: Not really, [I don't like being in the same class with Peter] 'cos sometimes he can be a pain, when he's good he's good but when he's bad I don't like him to be in my class because sometimes he tries to be funny but he's stupid and when the teacher is talking to us and Peter was shouting I couldn't understand what he was saying.

Pupil D: All the teachers gather round them and they shout and they speak loud and you're not able to concentrate.

Finally, others expressed their concern that disabled pupils may attract teachers' and others' attention at the expense of 'normal' children:

Pupil A: Like on parent's evening she [the teacher] might comment on their work and not ours 'cos, like, they're different and they [parents] know that we can do it but they don't know about them.

Pupil B: They get more attention [from the teachers], 'cos they might be stuck and the teachers are spending all the time with them.

In summary, the above discussion focused on the way children viewed and felt about the integration of disabled children. Children's accounts indicate the complexities and contradictions inherent in this process, projecting also the conflicting messages children are receiving from their wider social environment. In the same way as the children participating in Quicke and colleagues's (1990) study, the children of this study deployed every argument in the current debate for justifying their responses. Furthermore, my experience of analysing children's accounts of their attitudes towards integration shared something of Quicke's (1991) experience observing the discussions of sixth formers' attitudes to their working class roots:

In discussion groups it was observed that most participants were likely to use arguments based on both racist and tolerant themes, with some discussions going full circle, so that some people ended up expressing views which directly contradicted those used at the start of the discussion.

(Quicke 1991: 51)

Children's attitudes towards the integration process tended to be conflicting and confusing because they were ambivalent whether it was beneficial for disabled children to be educated in an ordinary school. This ambivalence preoccupied children's discussions and generated further controversies (i.e. defining integration, creating academic identities, locating 'the problems' and defining the notion of 'mixing'). In turn these areas were used to justify either the inclusion or the exclusion of disabled children from ordinary schools.

Even though it can be said that children were able to oscillate between an 'integrationist' and a 'segregationist' position regarding the education of their disabled peers, such a statement neither suffices nor helps to explain the implied unresolved controversies. The dilemma of whether it is beneficial for disabled individuals to be educated in ordinary schools was not invented by them. Perceptive children's comments on their dilemmas and conflicts also reflected the contradictions and tensions already existing in the wider social world. As Quicke has noted,

Children's views reflect those of the culture in which they are located . . .
Rather than adopting a romantic attitude about the natural goodness of
children, a more realistic view is to assume that attitudes towards disability and difficulty will be as diverse amongst children as they are in
society generally.

(Quicke 1985: 2)

The moral dilemma expressed by the children is a conflict at a societal level as
well. On the one hand it is connected with liberal cultural norms based on
notions of humanism, of helping and valuing disabled people. On the other
hand it is derived from the economic and political interests that focus on
standards, achievement and the smooth functioning of ordinary schools, thus
creating structures which assess disablement to mean lower status. Thus the
integrationist and/or segregationist opinions that children held were rationalizations intended to deal with a moral dilemma that was just as much cultural
as individual. But an examination of attitudes towards the process of integration, especially when *social* integration is the topic under discussion, also
requires an examination of the issues involved in forming relationships/friend-
ships between disabled and non-disabled children. This can be done only in
relation to the wider context of children's culture within which friendships are
of central importance. Thus the following chapter enters into the realm of children's culture in an attempt to explore the meaning children ascribe to their
interactional and perceptual patternings with their disabled peers.

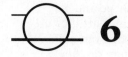 **6**

Disabled children and children's culture

The integration of disabled children into ordinary classrooms has been based partially on the assumption that contact between disabled and non-disabled individuals will result in them having constructive relationships with each other (Johnson and Johnson 1981; Stainback and Stainback 1981). Social integration has been perceived as a step towards providing interactional opportunities between disabled and non-disabled children, thus fostering greater acceptance and new perceptions upon which to form opinions and develop attitudes (Sheare 1974; Firth and Rapley 1990; Hellenbec and McMaster 1991; Kyle and Davies 1991). This assumption has been the focus of an increasing volume of research over the past four decades which has been directed towards the study of children's attitudes towards their disabled peers (Miller and Gibbs 1984; Shapiro and Morgolis 1988; Siperstein et al. 1988).

It has been reported that to a large extent the successful integration of disabled children depends on their interactions with and acceptance by their peers (Quicke 1985; Siperstein et al. 1988). In turn, it has been assumed that the way a child 'responds to his/her disability' can largely be shaped by the attitudes s/he first encounters in school and at home (Thomas 1982).

In Chapter 4 it was indicated that teachers perceived integration as an important mechanism for reducing prejudices by cultivating a social climate that would generate optimistic and positive interactions between disabled and non-disabled children. Despite, however, the great emphasis placed on the social aspect of integration, teachers could only offer some general assumptions to justify their beliefs. As the following accounts illustrate, teachers' responses to the question of how they perceived the social interactions between disabled and non-disabled peers were generally complex and diverse:

It's very difficult to answer, because I think in many ways young children change friendships so quickly that I would find it very difficult to say how our children interact.

They [children with special educational needs] actually go and play with other children . . . and the other children let them [but] they are not really bonded in special friendships. I don't think that our children [with special educational needs] really make best friends, do they?

I'm surprised really how tolerant and how caring the mainstream children are, but I'm not sure whether it's a kind of patronizing relationship where the mainstream children sort of patronize the less-able children.

That's a very difficult question . . . I think that the interaction would be very variable, quite frankly, for all sorts of reasons.

Sources of difficulty

Listening to teachers' responses, and at the same time trying to make sense of children's culture, I became increasingly aware of an issue identified by other researchers who have been involved in understanding children's cultural meanings. As Quicke *et al.* (1990: 127) indicate, 'we [researchers] were constantly aware of the possibility that both we and the teachers knew only a fraction of "what was really going on" amongst pupils'. At the same time, however, when exploring peers' attitudes towards the process of integration it involves an understanding of their attitudes towards their disabled peers which, in turn, cannot be separated from the wider children's culture which constitutes an important part of the social context in which their attitudes are located.

Central to this culture is the meaning that children ascribe to their complex and often volatile patternings of their interpersonal relationships. The exploration of children's meanings – regardless of whether we are referring to relationships among non-disabled or between disabled and non-disabled peers – is complicated (see Hargreaves 1972; Barnett and Zucker 1980) because, according to one view, each child's individual responses are affected by the wider social dimension (see Lynch 1987). As Hargreaves (1972: 7) has noted, 'the tension between the "social" and the "individual" is at its most acute in social psychology, which takes as its central focus interpersonal relationships'.

Also adults have difficulty in seeing children's culture, probably because children's culture is their own and thus 'not intended for adults' ears' (Opie and Opie 1959: 1). It is a culture which exists in its own right even though it is intimately related to and developed partly in response to adult's culture. Children position themselves within discursive practices learned from adult society in multiple and often contradictory ways (see Davies 1982). Even though they rely on the adult world because they have been located within structures designed by adults (i.e. children are taught about discursive practices through which they constitute themselves; see Davies 1989) they are not merely passive recipients of the messages they receive.

Despite this very important point it appears that often children's culture has been 'miniaturized' by adults or it has been perceived as a 'half-baked imitated version of adult culture' (Speier 1976: 99). When we try to explore the social context of children by viewing them as adults-in-the-making, we restrictedly perceive their activities as futile, random and less sophisticated, even though for them they include a high degree of structure and a complex purpose. For instance, regarding children's friendships, Gotmann metaphorically suggests that 'Children when beginning to make friendships must coordinate their efforts with all the virtuosity of an accomplished jazz quartet' (cited in Besag 1989: 76).

To begin with, we need to relate children's definitions of friendship to the particular structure within which children have been positioned. Children, because of their structural position, are among the most vulnerable groups in society, especially in those social contexts (i.e. family and school) which form most of their everyday life. That does not mean that they are powerless (even though that is the case in some circumstances); rather, it implies that they have to deal with social expectations, contradictions, ambiguities and evaluations that are not only externally imposed on them but which often can be potentially threatening for their own self-identity. They have to act within a social context where the conceptualization of their role includes a number of ambiguities:

> Children are important and unimportant, they are expected to behave childishly but are criticized for this childishness; they are supposed to play with absorption when told to play, and not mind stopping when told to stop, they are supposed to be dependent when adults prefer dependence and responsible when adults prefer that; they are supposed to think for themselves, but they are criticized for original solutions to problems.
>
> (Calvert 1975, cited in Pollard 1985: 65)

Speier (1976) has shown how the 'culture contact' of adults and children often restricts children's position in terms of conversational rights, especially when disagreements or arguments arise. This restriction is intensified in an educational environment where children are routinely judged on how well they can 'fit in' with the routines and activities which either the teacher or the institution develop in order to manage different situations. They have to comply with an official curriculum that they have little say over. As the following accounts indicate, this does not mean that they have nothing to say. Because they lack the power, though, to define what should count as the reality of schooling, their definitions of the situation have a lesser degree of stickability compared to teacher definitions:

> *Pupil A*: We want to do something that is more exciting, that we are more interested to do, but Mr G— just picks on something and he goes on from the books and we know every Monday we have to do this and that. I want to change the system. We should get a choice of what we want to do, like what topic we'd like to do. We should be able to choose.

Pupil B: Mr F— gives us hard work and expects us to do it. He expects us to do crosswords/

Pupil C: And sometimes he gets very annoyed. He expects us to do every-thing that he gives and if we do something wrong he shouts. I don't like it when he gets angry and starts shouting.

Pupil D: I'd like to change the way tables are. I would like the tables to be more closed together like Mr S— allows the children to sit wherever they want but in our class we have to sit boys and girls so that we can be quieter/

Pupil E: I would like in the class to have a more unisex colour. Now it's pink but I want a colour to suit both boys and girls, like green or red.

Within an educational environment the development of individual inter-ests, needs and desires can be regarded as impractical. This is partly because of the nature of the adult/teacher–child relationship, which is based to a large extent on an ongoing supervision and regulation of children's lives, and partly because of the limitations inherent in institutional organizations such as schools. Thus regardless of the way children view the situation, they are expected to accept it and to adjust their own lives to it. As Pollard sug-gests:

> Their success or failure [to do so] may have a great importance in terms of their identities and ultimately of their chances in life . . . The experi-ence of the children will vary, first according to their degree of acceptance of the teacher's curricular aims and second, if they do accept them, according to their ability to carry those aims out.
>
> (Pollard 1985: 84)

Of course, children's responses to their experience of schooling varied from child to child. The following exchange between two friends is indicative of the variation which exists among different children's experience of schooling; this variation is associated not only with the nature of the experience but also with the intensity of feelings involved:

Pupil A: I like school because as you get to a different stage and different age there are more things that you're learning . . . You can learn one thing from the television programme but you can learn much more from other things at school. I like the teachers/

Pupil B: Playtime is the best thing and dinner times. I like/

Pupil A: Yeah, I like both playtimes and dinner times. I don't like school holidays because you don't learn/

Pupil B: You're mad. If you are on holiday you can read your own books and sit on your chair and dream. You don't have to get up for sucking school.

Against this background, friends help children to cope with their structural positions in school and alleviate some of the threatening elements of school life. That does not mean that children's culture is unproblematic and conflict-free. Rather, it means that friendships in children's lives have a central place as a 'life-saving' response to the exigencies of the institution – fear, boredom, ritual routines, regulations and oppressive authority (see Woods 1977; Hargreaves 1982). They can often make all the difference between liking or loathing school. As Woods (1983: 96) notes, 'friendship groups form the structural basis of the child's extra-curricular life from a very early stage'. This childhood extra-curricular life serves as an antidote to the official system; its importance to children is as great as, if not even greater than, the formal social structure within which they have to spend a considerable part of their life. The importance of children's friendship groups can be demonstrated by the fact that the vast majority of children, when asked what they enjoyed the most from their school, indicated:

Pupil A: I like playing in the playground with my friends.

Pupil B: I like school because you can see and you can play with all your friends.

Pupil C: I like being at school because I meet most of my friends at school, while if I'm at home there are not many things to do. I'll be bored.

Pupil D: I like coming to school because I can see my friends, especially the ones who are far away.

The same responses were offered from the children identified as pupils with special educational needs when asked what they liked most about school:

Pupil A: I like playing police with my friends and arresting people who smash cars.

Pupil B: I like my friends. I like doing friends' letters.

Pupil C: I like it when people say they are your friends.

Pupil D: I don't like to leave school. I like playing with my friends in the playground and I like the green and the grass and the wind blowing the trees.

For children, friends are an integral part of school life. It is within these groups that children make sense of their experiences, and often they can establish new definitions of different schooling situations. In an exploration of how individual pupils define classroom situations, Furlong (1976: 163) has suggested that 'It is not enough to look at the individual on his [*sic*] own, for he's aware that his behaviour is a "joint action"; the others are taking part; that he's interacting.'

Thus the second function of friendship is to enable children to enter within that joint sphere, children's culture. Until they make friends they cannot participate. Their experience of being 'one of the crowd' (see Jackson 1968) can be reduced the moment they make friends and are enabled to participate in children's culture. As Davies maintains,

The fearfulness of this aloneness, the possibility of being outside children's culture, should not be underestimated when seeking to compre-
hend the children's understanding of the world of friendship . . . To be
alone in a new place without friends is potentially devastating. To find a
friend is to partially alleviate the problem.

(Davies 1982: 61–3)

It is during childhood that many children first experience loneliness (see Bell
1981). The centrality of being with your friends for friendship is illustrated
through the effects that not having friends can have:

Pupil A: If you don't have friends you'll be bored all the time . . . It's scary
to be alone.

Pupil B: [If I don't have friends] I'll feel sad because I would have to go
up and down and I would walk around with my hands in my pockets
and I would be alone and work and do things on my own and I don't
like that.

Pupil C: If you don't have friends you'll be sad and no one is going to play
with you . . . and you would just be looking around and everyone is
playing and you are alone.

Pupil D: [It is important to have friends] otherwise you'll be on your own
and you'll have nothing to do and you'll stand in the corner feeling
mad all alone. We need someone so that we don't feel sad and bored.

Because of the fear of being alone within an unknown crowd, 'being with
someone' becomes the core element of childhood friendship; while 'liking
someone' (from young children's point of view) has a specific instrumental
nature related to children's sense of vulnerability at school. In contrast to
adult assumptions (according to which the reason friendship develops is, for
example, that people like one another – see Wisman 1986), from a child's
point of view, especially during early childhood, friends are valued for their
physical accessibility, often their material and physical attributes. This does
not mean that liking does not constitute a part of childhood friendship; it
implies, rather, that it is not the most fundamental aspect of friendship. When
it is, children 'are clearer about the pragmatic nature of the liking than most
adults' (Davies 1982: 68).

A peer's willingness to be a playmate was valued as a friendly action; in turn
such a peer was referred to as being a friend. Within that framework a peer's
characterization as being or not being 'nice' was often based on the above criterion – for instance, 'She's nice because she plays with me.' This rule of childhood friendship was expressed in a higher degree and intensity by the Year 1
and 2 children, according to most of whom it was the 'violation' of this rule
by Nina, their peer with Down's Syndrome, that was partially the reason for
not wanting to be friends with her:

Pupil A: She's not nice . . . I don't like playing with Nina because she
doesn't want to play with me.

Pupil B: I don't like playing with Nina because she always runs off from the game. She doesn't sit to play with you.

Pupil C: I don't like her because she doesn't like me. She doesn't let me play with her.

According to the same logic,

Pupil D: I like Nina . . . She chases me and then she comes to find me and it's fun.

While such reasoning may be viewed from an adult's perspective as being a form of 'childish' behaviour based on irrational simplicity, for the children it constituted a basic rule of their culture because it was directly associated with one of their primary self-interests: entry to and maintenance of children's culture. Thus as Pollard maintains:

> The official system of the school, with its hierarchy, rules and particular criteria of evaluation, exists alongside the children's own social system, which may appear to be less formal but which also has its own hierarchy, rules and particular criteria of judgement.
>
> (Pollard 1985: 80)

It is these rules and particular criteria of judgement that render childhood culture enabling in one respect and constraining in another. On the one hand, by creating, understanding and manipulating these criteria children are able to construct their own reality/culture within adult-directed structures, which offers them a source of support and security in the interaction of the two cultures. On the other hand, to enter and maintain an enabling position within this reality demands a high degree of sophistication and conformity. That is because children's culture 'acts rather differently to provide norms, constraints and expectations which bear on its members' (Pollard 1985: 50). Implicit to this restraining aspect of children's culture lies the significance of friendship as serving many separate self-interests, rather than mutual interests. This applied even in the case of older children, who learn to think of interpersonal relationships as mutually reciprocal within which each person must begin to pay attention to the other's perspective. Even though adults might feel some revulsion to the selfishness of this idea, for children such egocentrism is necessary for self- and social survival; it is justifiable if we consider that during childhood, they come to learn some of the most fundamental social aspects of interpersonal relationships, including the preservation of identity and status within both peers' and adults' cultures. Thus it is not surprising that children view friendship as essentially an exchange relationship (see Thomas 1978).

Forming friendships: the first part of the friendship equation

> We come to like people we associate with because we associate with them, rather than because they are intrinsically likeable.
>
> (Davies 1982: 68)

The fact that proximity can lead to friendship has already been proposed by Homans (1951), who has suggested that the nearer two people are located in space, the greater the likelihood that they will come to like one another. This is so probably because the nearer together two people are, the greater the opportunity for interaction, while the more two people interact, the more they will like one another or at least the more they will come to know each other. The evidence of this research supports Homan's proposition in various ways.

First, children's perceptions of Sam (the girl in the picture) tended to be more negative than their perceptions of their actual peers with Down's Syndrome. This probably is closely related to the fact that the children 'came in contact' with Sam only once, while in their reality they had the opportunity to interact with their peers with Down's Syndrome on an everyday basis. Feelings of attraction are usually developed towards others with whom we have some close personal interaction defined by proximity. But within the research situation where a picture was used to initiate an interaction, the effect of proximity was not taken into consideration. In doing so, the use of the picture provided only one or, at most, two levels of interaction: that of a 'unilateral awareness' and 'surface contact' (Levinger 1974). Research concerning interracial acceptance has shown that the first level of interaction is influenced by the salience of race to the child (or, as in this case, disability), while responsiveness at the second level of contact would provide the lowest level or origin of acceptance (see Carter *et al.* 1980: 117–37). Thus excluding the opportunities offered by proximity simultaneously excludes the opportunity to become aware of other unique information about the individuals involved in shared experiences.

Second, in more general terms, the importance of proximity in interpersonal attraction was indicated by the fact that all children without exception referred to at least two people from their own class as being their friends. This does not negate the proposition that children tend to form friendships with other peers who are of the same age. Probably, the same-age factor is just one indicator of the high level of conformity in children's friendships. In many cases some of the friendship ties in the infants (Years 1 and 2) and in the junior level were left over from nursery where children met for the first time, thrown together by the force of circumstance. This finding confirms James's (1993) proposition that durability is an important feature in childhood friendships, not only for older pupils but for younger children as well.

Furthermore, propinquity and patterns of daily interactions may partly account for the close correspondence found between classroom seating plans and the patterning of children's friendships. For instance, in Years 1 and 2, 22 out of 29 children referred to someone they were sitting with as being their friends, while others referred to someone who happened to sit beside them in a previous class as friends. In the same way all 'resource children' referred to at least two other 'resource pupils' of the same class as being their friends, a likely result of these children's opportunity to spend a substantial amount of time together as a group sharing a number of different educational and social activities.

Finally, in Years 3 and 4, 20 out of the 27 children referred to at least one person from the same neighbourhood as being their friend. In some cases a chance meeting on the way to school was viewed by children as the first step towards friendship (see Davies 1982):

> *Pupil A*: I saw her [her best friend] at the school but we didn't talk or anything but she was living close to my house and one day when I was coming to school I noticed her and I waved to her and we came together to school and then we started to play together.

Neighbourhood propinquity seems to be important, not only because it is the place where children can meet for the first time before even entering the school community, but also because it offers children the opportunity to meet outside the school and to travel to and from school together, fostering in this way a sense of continuity and the strengthening of certain interpersonal relationships.

Also neighbourhood propinquity, while not being the most important element within childhood friendship, seemed to provide several opportunities for enriching interactions. Whereas this seemed to be a natural event for the majority of ordinary pupils, it was almost absent for all the so-called resource children except one. They were 'the ones who are coming by taxi', according to one child's definition of 'resource students'. According to another child, 'I haven't invited Peter [a peer with Down's Syndrome] to my house. I don't even know where he lives and he doesn't know where I live.' The importance of neighbourhood propinquity in friendships between disabled and non-disabled children is best illustrated by the following account from one of the teachers, who was also a parent of a disabled child:

> The children that are living close to their school they associate with at their homes as well. It's natural and that affects their friendship. While . . . I see that with my daughter . . . if you're living far away from your school environment, then it's very hard. There is a discontinuity in friendships. Friendships at home are artificially created. I mean if you have a birthday party who are you going to invite? Because the children that you spend half of your day with are at quite a distance from your house and transport has to be arranged, and yet sometimes they don't have the relationship in the neighbourhood to invite those children . . . The children should go to their local school . . . [otherwise] parents have to make special arrangements with local clubs if their child is not attending a local school. Because anyway these [disabled] children are regarded as the odd ones but you know, you need to belong . . . you belong to your family and then you belong to a wider family and then to your neighbourhood and then to your school and sometimes these [disabled] children find it difficult to identify themselves with any of these groups. They are in every place and it's not easy at all.

Proximity is of great significance in the creation of friendships, and to ignore its importance is to ignore a core element in the generation of interactions that can lead to the making of friendships. As James (1993: 219) maintains, 'Children's choices of their best friends are at least partially – if not substantially – affected by momentary factors like besides whom they are standing or sitting when they complete the [sociometric] test.'

The problem with this argument is that proximity, even though necessary, is by itself insufficient to explain why the physical placement of disabled children in ordinary schools does not necessarily lead to meaningful social integration as well (see Hoben 1980). To move from physical to social integration is to travel a long way, and involves a number of other complicated social parameters.

Forming friendships: the second part of the friendship equation

You see, really and truly, apart from the things anyone can pick up (the dressing and the proper way of speaking, and so on), the difference between a lady and a flower girl is not how she behaves, but how she's treated. I shall always be a flower girl to Professor Higgins, because he always treats me as a flower girl, and always will; but I know I can be a lady to you, because you always treat me as a lady, and always will.

(G. B. Shaw, *Pygmalion*, cited in Rosenthal and Jacobson 1968)

Understanding how people behave towards others necessitates an examination of how each party thinks about and perceives the 'other', as these two points of view are mutually interdependent (see Yuker 1988). Hargreaves (1972: 31) demonstrates convincingly that any analysis of human interaction 'clearly involves a consideration of the ways in which persons perceive one another. It is the perception of just who and what the other person is which steers one man's [*sic*] behaviour to another.'

The process of forming perceptions about an other is a complicated affair involving static and dynamic aspects. However, in any encounter there is a starting point; it is at this stage that appearance and physique are important criteria in impressionistic classification because they are associated with beliefs and assumptions upon which perceptions are based. As the following accounts indicate, appearance signals provide early social information which acts as an anticipatory signal to others, conveying clues that influence the formation of the other's perceived identity:

Pupil A: She [Claire] looks like a kind person . . . I notice it from her face, her mouth and her eyes.

Pupil B: Claire looks like a kind of bully. She looks like pushing everybody, calling names and pushing and fighting and swearing. I think Claire is good at bullying . . . Yeah, she's a bully because you can tell from her eyes and her face. She has a cruel face.

Pupil C: She [Claire] looks cleverer than Sam. She looks brighter. You can understand it from her face, from her eyes, from her smile.

Even when relationships are already formed, appearance seems to be a point of reference in descriptions of the other person. With younger children this phenomenon is intensified because, especially at the age of 6 to 7, children's descriptions of others tend to focus on simple traits and are orientated to the immediate and the concrete (Rogers 1978). For instance, when asked to describe their friends, children of Years 1 and 2 – but also older children – tended to concentrate on certain characteristics of physical appearance:

Pupil A: I like her. She's gorgeous. She's small, she has blonde hair and green eyes. I like it that she's small and has blonde hair. We have the same colour hair.

However, children refer to appearance signals not only because they concentrate on single and concrete elements in describing the others but also because they are undergoing the sociocultural training that makes sure that each generation acquires the ground rules and the associated values of what seems to be the 'appropriate social order of appearance'. As Thomas (1982) points out, these values are of course not simply applied to others, they are applied by the self to the self in the formation of the self-concept. Children, even from the age of 6, have already formed a subjective value of themselves in which body image, including visual appearance, is identified with self-image. Thus in the research interviews children claimed, among other things, that:

Pupil A: I look beautiful. I have a nice ponytail. I have beautiful hair. I'm lovely.

Pupil B: I look terrible. I look like a [unclear] . . . I am horrible.

Pupil C: I'm beautiful because I brush my hair every night. I have lots of girls behind me because I'm smart.

Pupil D: 'I've got short darkish brown hair and brown eyes. I've got a sun-colour. I'm pretty . . . [pause] I like to be pretty.

Pupil E: I'm ugly and if someone will say I'm ugly I'm going to call them names.

Often the 'I have' or 'I don't have' become 'I am' or 'I am not'. Appearance signals are of social importance because they are used to imply additional qualities and characteristics which in turn are used as the basis for inter-actional, emotional and evaluative responses. For instance, as a type of game all children were asked to describe Sam and Claire by using nine index cards with the following characterizations: 'naughty', 'clever', 'nice', 'has lots of friends', 'friendly', 'with good manners', 'without good manners', 'ugly', and 'beautiful'. According to the dominant pattern, children's connection of the different characterizations confirmed that a positively or negatively valued appearance can mean the attribution of other personal qualities and characteristics which follow the value direction of the physical characteristics (see Thomas 1982):

> *Pupil A*: Claire is beautiful, friendly, nice, clever, with good manners. Sam is ugly, without good manners, naughty.

> *Pupil B*: Claire is beautiful, with good manners, she's nice, clever, friendly and has lots of friends . . . Sam looks ugly, doesn't have good manners, she's naughty, she doesn't have a lot of friends. She's not nice.

The above 'physical attractiveness stereotype' is based on the wider sociocultural conventions that supply the ready-made typification that those who are beautiful are good – an assumption unlikely to have any foundation in fact (see Argyle 1975). In the same way, as a 6-year-old child blandly put it, there is the stereotype that 'Ugly people are rubbish.' However, as Booth (1985: 3) suggested, 'prejudices about talent and beauty are in all of us, and pressure for their removal may provoke deep-seated resistance'. Appearance, power, prestige and influence are important subsets of the dominant value-system in our society. It would be a mistake, however, to ignore that some aspects of the dominant value-system were challenged by some children:

> *Pupil A*: I have good manners, nice hair and beautiful teeth [two of his front teeth are missing] . . . [pause] No, I'm ugly and rich and I want to become a farmer [laughing].
> *Interviewer*: Why are you laughing?
> *Pupil A*: Because I'm ugly and I'm rich. I'm rich and you're thinking I'm going to pick, like, a big job and I just say a farmer, like a poor job.

Also, agreement on the meaning of symbols was by no means shared by everyone:

> *Pupil A*: She [Sam] is ugly and I don't want to have ugly friends/
> *Pupil B*: She's not ugly to everybody. She's not ugly to some people. There are some other people who may like her. I like her. She's nice with good manners.

> *Pupil C*: Sam is not very clever but she got good manners, she has a lot of friends, she's not naughty, she's not beautiful but she's not ugly.

Finally, for others the sociocultural meaning of symbols brought conflict:

> *Pupil A*: She's ugly with good manners, friendly, clever and nice.
> *Pupil B*: No, how can she be ugly and nice and friendly? You have to say ugly with no good manners/
> *Pupil A*: I think we should put the nice in and put the ugly out and put the friendly and the clever in . . . [pause] Well, she's ugly but you can be ugly, clever and nice at the same time!

These cultural meanings of appearance are of great importance in encounters with disabled people, not only because 'it is when trying to conform to such values that young disabled people feel most oppressed' (Quicke 1985: 159) but also because the sociocultural creation of difference begins from the values attached to appearance. Deviation in appearance is the first sign of attributing 'a handicapped identity'.

'She looks handicapped': a tale of 'us' and 'them'

'What is the function of this sensitivity to the appearance of others, this capacity to distinguish "normal" from "handicapped"?' (Thomas 1982: 16). How we come to attach social and functional meanings to physical variations is a process difficult to understand, but initial encounters with a disabled person illustrate the lessons we unconsciously learn in childhood:

Pupil A: She's ugly . . . She's not clever.
Interviewer: How do you know/
Pupil A: She's got this smile/
Pupil B: She looks thick.

Pupil C: She needs more help than Claire because she makes quite a lot of mistakes.
Interviewer: Oh I see. What makes you say that?
Pupil C: I'm just guessing. She just looks it.
Pupil D: She [Sam] is the opposite of the other one [Claire].
Pupil E: I think she looks like a disabled, like Patricia and Paul.

The Opies (1959) note in their *Lore and Language of Schoolchildren* that differences in appearances are of great significance to children in creating the vocabulary of distinctiveness, which becomes more subtle when it is used to provide an affirmation of 'a handicapped identity':

Pupil A: I think, like, because of her face that she has something like a bit of a mental something with her brain, 'cos you can tell those people when they have their face like that, like Spyros, it means that you have something mental. When there is something wrong with your brain then it shows on your face.

What seems to happen is that the visible signs of distinctiveness in appearance are the first challenges to the perceived appropriate social order of normalcy since they present an image physically different from the norm:

Pupil A: She looks funny. She has a big head and it sticks out and she's got big eyes. It looks as if her eyebrows have got more hair on, like, they're thicker and she's got that look.

Pupil B: She looks funny 'cos her smile is kind of funny and her eyes aren't straight. They're . . . this eye is bigger than that eye.

The cultural values attached to appearance-departures from the norm are acquired through an unconscious learning process involving perceptual comparisons which enable children to define others as 'exceptional', 'atypical' or 'not normal'. The vocabulary of distinctiveness is also a means of projecting that we belong to the unstigmatized, which is the first step in creating the story of 'us' and 'them':

> *Interviewer*: You think Sam looks a bit slow but Claire doesn't. How did you understand that?
> *Pupil A*: Because of her face/
> *Interviewer*: Her face? What about her face?
> *Pupil A*: Her eyes and how she smiles . . . Her face, it doesn't look exactly *like ours* would.
> *Interviewer*: Her face doesn't look exactly like/
> *Pupil B*: Other people's, *like normal people, like ours* but handicapped people would look like that [emphasis added].

> *Pupil C*: She's a resource student.
> *Interviewer*: How did you understand from the picture that Sam is a resource student?
> *Pupil C*: Because she doesn't look *like normal people*. Her head is lopsided and her eyes, like, look at her eyes and it is, like, look at her body. She's sitting like that. She's sitting funny. She's not straight [emphasis added].

> *Pupil D*: Is there something wrong with Sam? She doesn't *look like us* . . . She, she looks a bit like a resource person [emphasis added].

Deviations from the norm in physique and appearance are of course not simply statistical, neutral deviations – they posses value connotations when used to confirm a specific identity for the other. When this is taken with definitions of what it means to be 'disabled' or 'handicapped', appearance then becomes a factor which intensifies the social stigma of being disabled, thus enlarging the gulfs between 'us' ('the normal') and 'them' ('the disabled').

Defining disability

> Initial encounters between the disabled and others do not start from a neutral point, and the disabled person has to deal with definitions of himself and his disability previously and independently conceived by others.
>
> (Thomas 1982: 8)

The problem with the use of any label or category is that it focuses on one specific attribute at the expense of everything else about an individual. While the word 'disabled' had many meanings for the children in the study, its central function as a label was to distinguish the 'normal' from the 'not normal':

> *Pupil A*: [Disabled means] that you're not normal.

> *Pupil B*: They [disabled people] are not the same . . . [pause] they're not like us.

Pupil C: It [the word 'handicapped'] means that they're not like us. They have different faces and hands.

Pupil D: Disabled are people who cannot do things like normal people can do.

Pupil E: It [the word 'disabled'] means, like, you cannot do things that normal people like you and me and Julia and Kathreen can do.

Paradoxically, even though the attitudes towards what constitutes normalcy were very central and fundamental in maintaining social order, none of the children could explain what 'normal' means; as some of them claimed, 'It's just an English word.' It seems that our culture teaches us what the signs and symbols of normalcy are by indicating what is not normal, establishing in this way who is 'like us' and who is 'not like us'. Thus for children to be normal means to be 'like us', while not to be 'like us' means, as one child put it, that there is 'something wrong with you'. As Thomas writes:

> The notion that we use convenient conceptual packages when thinking about others is, of course, not new. Perceptions of national characteristics, racial groups and other 'outsider' minorities are part of our social education. They are built-in elements in our socialization. To 'be like us' is natural and normal, to be 'not like us' is foreign, unusual and abnormal.
>
> (Thomas 1978: 13)

Disability, in any form, seemed to be a violation of children's own priorities in relationships at this stage; it was not coincidental that children viewed disability in terms of what people so described could not do. As Quicke *et al.* (1990) note, children are more likely to refer to features such as 'talking' and 'movement' because in their perceptions of peer relationships competence in these areas is important. In children's words:

Pupil A: They cannot walk, they have to go on wheelchairs.

Pupil B: They don't listen very well and they do things that are very wrong.

Pupil C: They cannot talk properly.

Pupil D: They cannot do anything that I can do.

Pupil E: Disabled people cannot play or write properly.

An interesting finding was that older children often seemed to distinguish between 'disabled' and 'handicapped'. The word 'disabled' was used mainly when children referred to physically disabled children, as opposed to 'handicapped', which was used in describing mentally disabled people:

Pupil A: To be handicapped, it has to do with your brain but if you don't have a leg it has to do more with 'disabled'. Like there is a difference between 'disabled' and 'handicapped'. Someone is disabled when he has lost one of his senses or he has no leg or he uses a wheelchair. When you're going to the toilet you can see a sign saying disabled toilets and it shows a wheelchair, but 'handicapped' is more like someone who is mentally ill. It has to do with brain damage.

Pupil B: My mum is disabled and it means, like, you know, handicapped people have trouble with part of their face but disabled people have a problem with part of their body, like their arms and their legs.

Pupil C: I grew up thinking that disabled is someone sitting in a wheelchair or having problems with their legs but now I know there are handicapped people as well who are not able to understand things because their brain doesn't work properly. Like, when you get older, about your age, they still have the brain of [someone aged] 10. Their brains are not like ours – it [their brain] stopped growing.

Often the label 'handicapped' evoked more derogatory stereotypes projecting some of the gross prejudices surrounding mentally disabled people:

Pupil A: They [handicapped children] bit their parents.

Pupil B: Handicapped are worse than disabled, because handicapped never learn even when teachers are doing everything.

Pupil C: Handicapped people are bad and they're going to the special school to learn how to be kind.

Pupil A: Handicapped people don't learn things because they cannot write and read and when they grow up they will rob shops. I know someone who is handicapped and he robs shops now because he doesn't know what/
Pupil B: No, no, Anastasia. I/
Pupil A: Because he cannot understand what anything means. He didn't learn anything at school and he didn't understand what letters mean and he cannot sign up/
Pupil B: No, Anastasia, I know that man but he doesn't rob shops.

Pupil F: We don't make friends with handicapped because . . . they might get killed . . . They might be silly and they go to the doctor and they can take you on their motorbike somewhere and kill you.
Pupil G: Yeah, like kidnappers. My mum said that people kidnap you and take you in a car and they can take you away . . . I have some people next to my house and they're handicapped and they take drugs because they're silly.

Words used to describe people can be both a manifestation and a determinant of an attitude. Children had learned to view disability as an attribute of the individual – 'they have something wrong inside' – with no acknowledgement of it being the outcome of a relationship between people with an impairment and the rest of society. According to this general deficit view, a handicapped identity is conferred upon a person by reason of his/her physical/functional difference. The medical model is a very well-known example; it treats disability as a defect in the individual, and his/her symptoms as the signs of an underlying cause of disability.

Such perceptions are likely to influence the formation of interpersonal relationships; their implied values will be expressed in friendship acts and deeds. As Thomas (1978) has suggested, children's definitions of disability and disabled individuals gradually develop to have personal and social consequences for both disabled and non-disabled persons, as well as for their interactions, because such definitions rigidify preconceived identities. For instance, disability was strongly connected with notions of dependence – a belief legitimized by the perceived identity of disabled people as those 'who are not able to do things like ordinary people can':

Pupil A: They need people to help them because they cannot do things.

Pupil B: I cannot imagine how they will be when they will grow up. I think that they will need someone to live with them and help them like a guardian.

Pupil C: [Handicapped children] are the children who need help, like with the work in school because they grow up with problems.

Pupil D: They need help because they don't know what to do.

Pupil E: She [Sam] cannot brush her teeth 'cos she doesn't know what to do. She doesn't know how to eat. Her mum has to feed her.

Often disability, especially mental disability, was extended to cover the whole personality and humanity of the person:

Interviewer: We talked a lot about Sam but we didn't talk a lot about Claire.

Pupil A: Probably she [Claire] would get embarrassed if she was talked about a lot.

Interviewer: You think so?

Pupil A: Yeah, because, like Sam might not know the meaning of the word embarrassed and she won't get embarrassed.

Someone who looks different is perceived as both thinking and feeling different than other human beings. There were, however, children who viewed an impairment as part of the individual with some functional consequences; people with impairments did not therefore have to belong to a different human category:

Pupil A: They [disabled people] are like us but there are some things that they cannot do . . . so if the teacher has to teach them a game she has to show them what to do.

Pupil B: They [disabled people] are ordinary people apart from the fact that they have lost one of their senses, like hearing, or some of them may have lost two senses, like they cannot see and they have lost their hearing senses but when you lose a sense then you get another sense better/

Pupil C: You add to your senses like you cannot have an extra sense but you can add to your other senses like you could feel things more or you can see more than what we can do.

If it can be assumed that a person chooses for his/her friends those who he/she perceives to be like him/herself in some significant respects (see Ball 1984; see also Hargreaves 1972), then this basic perceptual division between 'us' and 'them', as reflected in the majority of children's accounts, constitutes an additional hindrance to smooth interactions between disabled and non-disabled children.

In an educational context the distinction between 'us' and the 'them' is being strengthened, especially for mentally disabled children, because schools 'are one of a very few remaining public interactional spaces in which people are still engaged with each other in the reciprocal, though *organizationally patterned*, labour of producing meaning – indeed, the core meaning of self-identity' (Wexler 1992: 10, emphasis added). The creation and meaning of self-identity in a school context is strongly associated with academic competence, which is not only a means for surviving but is associated with values that form the basis for the evaluation of both the self and the other's self. At school, 'to be clever' is significant because this becomes an important criterion upon which school-structured identities are officially formed. In turn, these school-structured identities influence the creation of friendship ties because what happens within the classroom setting influences what happens outside the classroom (Ball 1984; Pollard 1985; Roffey *et al.* 1994).

School-structured identities: 'ordinary' and 'resource' students

Academic achievement was not mentioned by any child as being a characteristic of friendship ties, but it was a source of feedback in the development of each child's identity. The subjective valuations that children had formed about themselves, even from the age of 6, in addition to body image, were also based on their sense of competence in academic terms:

Pupil A: I'm quite intelligent. I'm good at English and stories. I'm quite good at English and stories. I'm quite good at tests and I take high marks. I want to be a doctor or something involved with the hospital. I'm quite ambitious.

Pupil B: I would like to be more cleverer than I'm now. I know that I can be more cleverer [but] I always get into trouble because I do practical jokes.

Pupil C: I want a lot of help. I'm not a very good student. I want some help with writing . . . Spelling makes me angry.

As Pollard maintains,

> to learn in lessons is not an interest-at-hand simply by virtue of the need to cope with the particular situation. It is linked to the maintenance of self-image, to enjoyment, to stress avoidance and to dignity – facets which, though experienced with immediacy, accumulate over time into more established identities.
>
> (Pollard 1992: 89)

Children, however, do not develop a 'conception of self' until after a conception of others has been acquired (see James 1993: 216). They learn about their status at the institution only in relation to the other's status. Someone is 'slow' or 'slower' only in relation to someone else. Perceptual comparisons cannot be made unless there are some criteria of measurement and other people to compare the self with:

> *Pupil A*: I like maths. We have to do three books at maths and some people are doing book 1, others do book 2. I do book 3.

Academic achievement was an integral piece in the whole puzzle of developing the image of the other. Children were aware of what teachers expected of them and what they expected from other children. They knew who was famous in the class in terms of academic achievement, who had more stars and why, who had the most or the least house-points and what such award-systems meant. Often they were just too aware of teachers' evaluation systems, expectations and even preferences:

> *Pupil A*: Smith [is the most popular] because she's clever. She's known to get the higher grades in the class. I like Smith but Mr F— treats her like a kind of pet and I don't like this. If someone will do something that he didn't suppose to do it then he says 'I am sorry' but Mr F— says 'You're stupid'. If Smith do the same thing and is in trouble, it is OK for her. He let her go off and he's always checking her work to make sure she's not making any mistakes. If someone has missed a lesson like with Philips that he missed this medieval thing, Mr F— told him to go and take the notes from Smith. He never trusts anybody else with the notes, and if he doesn't remember something again he asks Smith.

> *Pupil B*: Paula is the least famous because she comes with a taxi because she lives far away and sometimes she has forgotten to bring some stuff but because she was in a rush she forgot and Mr G— always [he's] asking her the hardest questions and if she doesn't know then he's always shouting at her and it's not fair.

Through classroom experience each child comes to know who is the 'teacher's pet' and who is 'bright/clever'. This awareness influences their friendship groups and the nature of their interactions because as Pollard (1992) has shown, learning is of significant interest in the development of a particular identity, for such ability is part of the competence required of group members (see also Quicke and Winter 1994). The presumed identity for children defined as being the 'resource pupils' was that they were 'always slow' and 'not very brainy', either because of their disability (as far as older children were concerned), or because of their behaviour (the younger children). 'Resource pupils'' perceived identity had become so firmly established that it had come to be regarded as a stable element of their self-concept. In older classes, 'resource pupils' were not even included in those groups of ordinary children perceived by their peers as being 'slow'. They had been attributed a group or subcultural identity which by definition had a status subordinate to majority interests and which restricted their entry into certain roles. They were viewed as 'a separate group' or as a 'quarter of the class'; they were different from the rest of the class because they were 'the special needs children'. Such a school-structured identity was just one among many ways of reinforcing the story of 'us' and 'them'; it hindered meaningful relationships in the classroom, even when activities were ostensibly constructed to include all children.

The significance of academic competence is mainly associated with the official curriculum and its socio-educational values, such as the premium based on academic achievement which, in turn, derives from the purposes of the school. However, its influence on the formation of relationships is just too important to be ignored (see Hargreaves 1967; Wexler 1992) even in a primary school setting. It was not coincidental that older children expressed a concern about whether Sam would like to be in an ordinary school on the basis that she would have to deal with 'some brainy students' who might 'torment' her by calling her 'stupid' because 'she is not as brilliant as them'. But the notion of competence affects children's culture in many ways; the social consequences of the privileging of academic achievement are one example. In fact, disabled children have to deal with a number of culturally established expectations that cause difficulties in forming interpersonal relationships; their problems are doubly exacerbated because such expectations directly serve the interests-at-hand of those who create the expectations in the first place.

The cloak of competence: behaviour in context

While children's reactions to the photograph of Sam showed that appearance was indeed of primary importance in their evaluations of the other, it was clear that behaviour and functionalism ranked high as a hindrance to smooth interactions between them and their actual disabled peers. However, 'When judgements are made on socio-behavioural grounds, then the social context in which they are formed becomes critical in understanding how people are categorized' (Thomas 1978: 15).

Several researchers (Goodman *et al.* 1972; Peterson and Haralick 1977) suggest, as did many of the teachers interviewed, that younger children are more 'accepting' of disabled children than are older children. The findings of this study suggest that the issue is much more complicated. It was found that the younger children expressed more rejecting attitudes towards Nina, their peer with Down's Syndrome, than did the older children. At the same time, however, in the playground it seemed that a child with Down's Syndrome was involved with his/her peers to a greater extent than the children with Down's Syndrome at the junior level. This apparent contradiction raises some interesting issues. Of course the different personalities and social skills exhibited by these different children with Down's Syndrome influenced substantially the frequency, nature and quality of their interchanges with non-disabled peers. However, the way children of different ages conceptualized the notion of friendship – along with their self-needs and the structures of their games – all played their part. I acknowledge that types of friendship and self-needs are not necessarily contingent on age and that a simple hierarchical developmental model of friendship cannot be sustained. As James (1993: 216) indicates, 'there may be a considerable blurring of categories of "friend" and any individual child might be at different stages of friendship with different people'. At the same time, however, 'there are complex interactions between cognitive development (levels of understanding), moral development (ideas about right and wrong in relation to others) and learning experiences which affect social development' (Roffey *et al.* 1994: 121); these in turn change the conceptualization of friendship and the interests that friendship comes to fulfil.

Early childhood is the most significant period in the formation of identity, even though the sense of identity which is produced by such early socialization will continue to develop through other experiences (see Pollard 1985: 242). However, the younger the child, the more significant these experiences are likely to be. One of these experiences is the sense of vulnerability that young children feel when they are forced to rely on their resources to deal effectively with the crowd of a school playground. In attempts to reduce their feelings of fear and uncertainty children in the study were willing to be friends with every peer who expressed a willingness to be a playmate. Often that included the supplementary rule that the other is willing to play 'what I want to play', which is connected with the instrumental view of friendship in terms of how enjoyable and rewarding a particular relationship can be. Rejection was often a consequence of the other not satisfying this interest; this was mentioned frequently by children in justifying why they did not want to play with their peer with Down's Syndrome.

Peers were characterized as being 'nice' or 'not nice' mainly according to their willingness to be or not to be playmates. Such a willingness seemed to be an indication of 'liking', which reduced the fear of the other hurting the self. The ground rule was that 'no one wants to be your friend when you're fighting and kicking'. Among young children the term 'friend' usually referred to what they conceived of as 'friendly behaviour'. Conversely children often rejected as friends those whose behaviour was interpreted and classified as unfriendly. Any mild 'aggressive' behaviour such as kicking, thumping, pinching – even though a frequent occurrence in childhood relationships – was classified as unfriendly; it not only strengthened the fear about the other but also implied that the other was transmitting feelings of disliking.

For instance, after extensive discussions between Nina and me, as well as careful observations of Nina in the playground, it seemed that pinching or kicking was a way for her to initiate an interaction: mainly, Nina pinched a child and he/she chased her. Indeed, often such actions were the beginning of interactive activities. These different 'ways of communication' expressed by the peer with Down's Syndrome were often misunderstood by the other children, who felt such actions indicated feelings of 'disliking'. Relevant to this observation is Hargreaves's (1972) proposition that we tend to like people who we think like us; thus if a child is given information (such as kicking, thumping, pinching) that another child does not like him/her, then the first child will tend not to like the second.

Simultaneously, children were testing ways of dealing with conflict and differences: either they called an adult to solve the problem or they tended to ignore children who behaved in ways they didn't like; the most frequent response was to reciprocate. Participant observations and discussions with children, both younger and older, confirmed Davies's (1982) proposition that children speak more often of negative rather than positive reciprocity:

> *Pupil A*: I like him to be nice to me, not to fight me because that will make me fight as well.

> *Pupil B*: She [Nina] pushes people because she likes to and then she kicks me and I kick her.

> *Pupil C*: [If a friend won't talk to me] I will ignore her and get away and go and play with somebody else.

Negative reciprocity is an important rule in childhood culture because, according to children's perceptions, there is the proposition that 'I am a mirror to you which provides you with my perception of your behaviour towards me', which is somehow different from Cooley's proposition of the looking-glass self (see Davies 1982: 76). As Davies indicates, 'The unquestioning way in which reciprocal acts are engaged in clearly involves a controlling element, though the children do not necessarily accept "control" as their motivation' (p. 83).

Children learn, through the responses of others, that their own behaviour has consequences. It is this very basic rule of reciprocity and its functions that give the impression that children's relationships are unstable and involve a substantial amount of quarrelling. Quarrelling and fights originating out of the reciprocity rule were the strategies used by children for dealing with the delicate balance of the power games that form a part of relationships (see Davies's analysis of the notion 'contingency friends', which was also confirmed by this study). But the reciprocity rule meant that mentally disabled children seemed to be quite vulnerable, not only because they often were not able to understand fully these cultural contexts but also because their ways of initiating interactions were easily misunderstood by their peers. Disabled children's behaviour (in this case, Nina's behaviour) was doubly misunderstood: children had limited information on and comprehension of disability issues in general; and they were unable or found it difficult to find a satisfactory explanation for the other's often unpredictable behaviour in particular.

Thus children often focused on the behaviour solely, using this as the basis for identifying the other as being 'naughty' or 'disabled'. Their limited knowledge of what the second label meant contributed to the creation of less 'tolerant' and 'accepting' approaches towards their peer with Down's Syndrome, because her actions both puzzled them and challenged their emerging concepts of acceptable patterns of behaviour.

There is, however, another side of the coin. While children expressed quite negative responses towards their peer with Down's Syndrome, with the vast majority of them claiming that they 'were not Nina's friend because . . .' for a number of behavioural reasons, in the playground children were often seen to play with her. There are a number of explanations for this contradiction. First, younger children are at the beginning of the process of creating self-presentation techniques (see Goffman 1971), so in discussions with them they tended to use their 'authentic' voices in talking about the other, even when their descriptions tended, from an adult perspective, to sound negative or even cruel. As they got older, they appeared more concerned about the version of self that they wished to present to the other – i.e. the researcher – and thus were constrained in expressing authentically their thoughts and opinions. Second, it is well known that at one moment children claim that they are not friends with someone while at the very next moment they can be seen playing happily together:

Pupil A: They [friends] are kind to you.
Pupil B: Sometimes they're not because once Pam hit Susan.
Interviewer: And what did you do, Susan?
Pupil C: I told it to Miss and then I became friends with Pam.

Even though at one point children – in a discussion – claimed that they would not like to play with Nina, in the playground they were seen to be involved in interactions with her. This is also associated with the nature and the structure of their games, which tend to be more flexible and inclusive compared to the structures, hierarchical rules and roles involved in the dynamics of older children's games. Of course every encounter exhibits sanctioned orderliness arising from obligations fulfilled and expectations realized (see Goffman 1961). However, it was easier for every child at different times to gain access to younger children's games, such as chasing, skipping, and playing in the igloo. Children were able to change from one game to another, often being involved with different peers for the duration of a single break-time. This playground context was different from the one observed at the junior level, in which gaining social acceptance within a group or forming deeper relationships was related to the more established norms of behaviour within the group. Here children, in order to gain access and maintain an enabling position within the different groups, had to acquire the values, attitudes, language and images of the group – processes that include conformity and other highly sophisticated strategies.

As children grow up they learn that 'friendship' is a very complex social relation; the factors that shape the patterns and courses of their friendships extend further than the willingness of someone to be a playmate – although for the older children such a willingness was still of great importance. For them, it was one thing 'to have' friends and another 'to be' friends (as these terms have been defined by James 1993).

The dynamics involved in the formation of 'being friends' with someone are multidimensional and have been analysed extensively by other researchers (see Foot *et al.* 1980; McGhee and Chapman 1980; Davies 1982; James 1993). The difference, however, between 'having' and 'being' friends is that the latter involves complex manoeuvres of maintaining the friendship, a great deal of emotional and self-investment, relations between the self as the 'ego' and the friend as the 'alter ego', as well as more sharing and participative interactions. This differentiation is significant because, according to the dominant pattern in the study, disabled children experienced the context of 'having' friends rather than 'being' friends with non-disabled children. For instance, the other children viewed them more as contingency friends, as someone who keeps you company and plays with you when you have broken up with your 'friends'. Most of the disabled children were not socially isolated through an absence of company or even an engaging social network – their isolation stemmed from the absence of these more complex and at the same time intense and mutually participative interactions involved in the context of 'being' friends. They were perceived as friends but not 'proper' friends.

Notions of competence, functionalism and behaviour were used as reasons for explaining why disabled peers were not 'proper' friends or why they were excluded from game contexts. The list of functional difficulties that children referred to was quite long. Implicitly, mentally disabled children were often rejected because they did not fulfil expectations and culturally defined goals as well as the approved means of reaching them. In more subtle ways the rejection of disabled children was associated with an important element of childhood culture: the acquisition of status. As Pollard (1992: 49) maintains: 'Status . . . to some extent . . . cuts across the questions of friendship relations and of social competence and in a sense it summarises their social outcome.' Furthermore, Davies (1982) has shown that how and why who can do what to whom in a particular situation depends on their status.

Status: a primary self-interest

Beyond the struggles of 'having' and of 'being' friends lay the primary concern of presenting an acceptable image of the self in the public demonstration of sociality which playtime represented. One of the many functions that 'friendship' served was to provide the means for the creation of a satisfactory image of personhood. In turn, beyond the concern of children to be seen as full and competent members of their group lay the concern of obtaining a specific status. This was an important means of protecting their self and surviving the variety of situations which they encountered at school. The social position of the self, however, was influenced not only by the amount of friends that someone had and his/her ability to present a competent self but by the image that had been attributed to his/her friends as well. To be liked by or to be friends with the leader of the football team or with someone who was considered as being 'naughty and nasty' played an important role in the creation of one's own image and, consequently, on the formation of friendships with others. One child, Jim, described his experience: 'I think I don't have lots of friends because sometimes when I play with Tom and another friend comes up and I say I play with Tom then he just goes away and finds another friend and you lose him.' In the group discussion in which Tom was present, Jim explained that 'they [the others] do that because I think they don't want to interrupt things'. However, in a private discussion that I had with Jim he explained to me that no one wanted to be with him when he was with Tom because Tom was considered by the others as being 'nasty'. In fact from participant observations, discussions with the other children and the sociometric devices employed it was noted that Tom was both socially and emotionally isolated. According to the teacher, 'he's a very strange boy. He cannot form relationships with other children. He doesn't know how to mix with people. He shows off a lot. He hits people . . . he's shouting and screaming.' As regards forming friendships, Jim knew that his friendly relationship with Tom had consequences for his own position within his peer group. Nevertheless, he continued to be friends with Tom because: 'I know he's shouting a lot but there is another thing with him as well. He has two sides: one soft inside and one hard from the outside. I found that out myself. When he's in the fighting mood and the ball comes to his chest he doesn't say "Ouch" but when he's in the soft mood and the ball comes to his chest he says "Ouch".'

While Jim's explanation is revealing, at this point it is more relevant to note that children, even from a very young age, put into practice the old adage that 'You can judge someone by the company they keep.' Being friends with disabled individuals influences a child's 'image' and 'status' because s/he is obliged, by the others' assumptions, 'to share something of the discredit of the stigmatized person to whom they are related'. As Goffman maintains, 'The tendency for a stigma to spread from the stigmatized individual to his [sic] close connections provides a reason why such relations tend either to be avoided or to be terminated, where existing' (Goffman 1963: 43). In children's words,

> *Pupil A*: [I don't want to be friends with Sam] because she has a big head and she looks silly. If I play with people with big heads someone may laugh at me.
>
> *Pupil B*: I don't think that people like to go with handicapped because other people will pick on them.

Pupil C: Some people think they're tough and disabled people are weak so they don't want to be seen with them.

Pupil D: You don't want people to see you with handicapped people. They'll pick on you.

But what seemed to be a barrier for some was an inspiration for others.

A process of redefining?

Discussions with children revealed that 'feeling sorry for' was a frequent response offered, mainly by girls, in explaining the reasons for forming friendly relationships with disabled peers. In some cases such a reason was surrounded by conflict and confusion:

Pupil A: He [Spyros] comes up to you and asks you if you want to play cowboys and Indians and you feel so sorry for him that you play with him. So if he would come up to me and Judi and ask us if we want to play with him [we would normally say] 'Yes, we are going to play with him.' We would not say that we want to play another game.

Interviewer: Why do you feel sorry for him?

Pupil B: You look at him and you feel like we better play with him because he's alone and he has nothing to do and then you think that if you were Spyros and you were seeing yourself lonely and you could not help it and you feel, like, sorry and you feel, like, sad about him so you go and play with him/

Pupil A: There are a lot of people who play with him because they feel sorry. I don't feel sorry for him, because these [disabled] people are born and the determination that people have got to actually become a normal person it's incredible. I'm treating him like a normal person and I don't feel sorry for him.

It is a controversial judgement whether there is 'anything wrong with "feeling sorry for"' (see Quick *et al.* 1990: 121). The important issue here is that no child offered this as a reason for explaining his/her friendly relationships with other ordinary peers. On the other hand, while 'feeling sorry for' can be 'the first step towards genuine empathy and understanding' (Quicke *et al.* 1990: 121) it is probably one of the reasons, whenever friendly relationships existed, why disabled peers were perceived as friends but not 'proper' friends.

The process of redefining involves other issues and questions. As Taylor and Bogdan suggest:

People who are involved in accepting relationships eventually take them for granted, something that does not require an explanation. In fact, asking people about why they have the relationships may evoke expressions of bewilderment, impatience or even disgust. This tells them that the person asking the question regards the relationship as something abnormal, that needs to be explained.

(Taylor and Bogdan 1989: 27)

As the following account illustrates, in already-formed relationships between disabled and non-disabled children the 'disability' becomes less central to the relationship while the shared activities are of more importance:

Interviewer: Do you have any disabled friends?
All together: No.
Pupil A: Oh, no, Anastasia. Peter is my friend. He's in my class. I play football with him . . . Once we went to a fair and then we went to his home and it was late. Peter asked his mum 'Can Charly stay here tonight?' and his mum told him no but his dad said yes and I slept over there. We woke up the next day and we played football.
[At another phase of the discussion]
Pupil A: It was a disco here at school. His [Peter's] mum said he couldn't go because no one could pick him up, no one could take him to the disco and I got up early in the morning, I got Graham [another friend] and we said we'll take Peter with us . . . [the discussion evolved around the disco party which concluded as being 'good fun' and 'great'].

Children who had formed inclusive relationships with their disabled peers related to the other as a person rather than as a 'stereotype', by focusing more on the humanity rather than the 'disability' of the person. This constituted the sentiment or the motivation for entering into such relationships such as those mentioned in response to general questions such as 'Who is your best friend?':

Pupil A: I'll talk about me and Peter. He's quite nice as a friend, the only problem is that he's kissing my hand . . . Sometimes he comes and starts pulling a funny act to make me laugh. He cheers me up. He's kind and funny . . . He's always there for me so I'm there for him. He says in his language 'You are my friend' . . . Now I can understand what he's saying.

Pupil B: [Spyros] he's my very best friend. First I didn't like him but he liked everyone, even people who fighted him. He's very friendly . . . Sometimes I help him and he helps me. I never fell out with him.

Pupil C: He's [Peter] my second best friend. He's a very, very, very, funny guy . . . He likes football and wrestling.

While the patterns of such accepting relationships varied, their central element was that the other was viewed in terms of his/her contribution to the relationship and his/her positive attributes rather than his/her difficulties. This approach seemed to be qualitatively different from the more dominant passive view that was to be found in other relationships between disabled and non-disabled children:

Pupil A: You know these Greek dances that you showed us? We help him to learn them and we dance together/
Pupil B: And he shows us how to catch the ball.

Pupil A: He can catch it good/
Pupil B: He catches the ball better than we can.
Pupil A: When someone is after us then he [Spyros] helps us. If someone is kicking me he goes and puts him down.

The above children were aware that their friend was 'different', but difference was given positive meaning, 'forming part of the explanation of the unique value to that person as an intimate' (Bogdan and Taylor 1987: 38):

Pupil A: Sometimes he's [Peter] hilarious, like dead funny being with him. You can laugh all the time . . . He and Patricia pretend that they want to get married and me and my friends we were pretending that we were priests and they kissed, and then they got into the car and we went around the school but we all pretend. Like we pretend that we are in a disco or that we are in an aeroplane. They have a wild imagination, they can imagine us that we are drivers . . .

On the one hand, the relationship was described in terms of liking and enjoying the company of the disabled peer (see Strully and Strully 1985; Perske and Perske 1988; Gold 1994). On the other hand, the 'disability' – while being acknowledged – was not seen as the central organizing factor around which explanations of the relationship were constructed. The following short account is quite illustrative of this different approach to interactions with disabled individuals. The discussion is based on the idea of a hypothetical birthday party and the activities that children (males) will do at this party after picking one of the two girls in the picture:

Interviewer: Let's say that you're Sam's friends and/
Pupil A: No, I won't be her friend. She's handicapped/
Interviewer: You don't want to be her friend because she's handicapped.
Pupil A: Yeah.
Pupil B: Yeah.
Pupil C: [impatiently and with a raised tone of voice] No, no, no. I don't like to put people off like that. I don't like to pick on people like that. I think I would pick them both.

Such an approach can become the basis of forming an enabling social identity of the other, and includes sensitivities and talents that labels such as 'handicapped' and 'disabled' cannot capture. If there is to be a concluding remark for this chapter then Goode's (1984) suggestion is significant. He has shown that in order to understand how 'handicapped' identities are socially produced it is necessary to reflect upon the way(s) different people perceive the same disabled person. Or as a child put it:

Pupil A: They don't really know her [Nina, a child with Down's Syndrome] that much.
Interviewer: What do you think they have to know about her?
Pupil A: That she's not horrible. She's nice and kind.

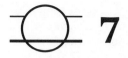 **7**

Conclusion

> For every complex issue there is a simple answer, and it is wrong.
> (H. L. Mencken, quoted in Zigler and Hodapp 1986)

It is important to remember that this study was taking place at a time when the education system in England and Wales was – as it still is – undergoing a transformation brought about by remorseless government pressure to impose change on schools and teachers via the introduction of numerous policies and innovations. These have covered all aspects of educational provision, policy and practice, including the values that underpin them. The dominant characteristic of this period has been the government's extensive efforts to introduce a centralized competitive market system for the supply of educational services, which has resulted in changes to the governance, content and outcome of schooling. The '"free-market" economic ideology and its "laissez-faire" social philosophy' (Carr and Quicke 1990: 434) have increasingly demanded that schools become more responsive to the economic needs of society in general and the labour requirements of industry in particular. Also a framework has been created within which 'the rhetoric of differentiation both within and between schools to cater for individual abilities and interests was deployed to "raise standards" and to establish criteria to facilitate parental choice' (Carr and Quicke 1990: 435). At this point in the historical development of education the present study has attempted to explore the question of attitudes towards integration and, particularly, to locate the question of inclusive education within the wider context of a changing educational system.

Inclusive principles and the new education era

The findings of this study support the view that integration has become a contentious issue. Nearly all the teachers showed that their attitudes towards the process of integration were confused and often conflicting – the notion of integration had no coherent meaning for them. Its meaning was, rather, to be found in the context and purpose of its use being contingent on several educational (im)practicalities, while a whole range of practices that were called integration were actually expressions of segregationalist mentalities. Teachers' contradictory views of the 'special' and 'integration' – as well as the wider social structures in which teachers work – seemed to perpetuate the vicious circle of the exclusion of a particular group of children. The ideological and practical themes that were raised in teachers' discourses about integration revealed the degree and nature of the barriers that need to be overcome if praiseworthy ideals are to become reality.

It has been emphasized that teachers' willingness and commitment to promoting inclusive priorities were influenced to a great extent by *the educational context*. In other words, teachers are policy-makers but their policy/practices are contingent on the institutional and wider ideological conditions within which they apply them.

According to teachers, teaching is not what it used to be. They did not experience the same degree of enjoyment and fulfilment as they had in the past because the recent economic and political changes tended to undermine their morale and motivation. The new demands were perceived as threatening some of their most fundamental interests-at-hand, such as satisfaction, workload and autonomy.

The insights offered in this account must not be taken to imply that these teachers felt that all the changes taking place were unacceptable or that a national curriculum was not important. What they found objectionable was the dogmatic nature and imposition of many of these changes and their resulting detrimental effect on teachers' self-esteem and job satisfaction.

Teachers felt that they were being threatened by the introduction of a value-for-money mentality with regard to educational planning and practice. They found themselves within a context where the defining principles of professional commitment were changing. Thus they felt that they had to intensify their efforts so as to preserve a balance between the demands of political and market forces and the demands of children: demands that were difficult to reconcile.

The frantic pace, extreme scope and breadth of the legislative powers used by goverment, combined with the confusion often engendered by the new demands and practicalities/technicalities, encouraged many teachers to adopt the strategy of 'just coping' with the situation. But as Elliot (1990) has indicated, there comes a point when such a strategy might no longer be fair either to pupils or to teachers.

The pressures of 'coping' or 'managing their time' left teachers with little physical and psychological space and energy for developing the most fundamental element of teaching: reflecting upon their own practice (see Mittler 1992). Besides, the new ethos of commercialism is not sympathetic to the development of teachers' powers of self-reflection; teachers have been criticized for 'their failure to maintain standards, discipline and provide school leavers with the appropriate attitudes and skills necessary for competing effectively in the market place' (Vlachou and Barton 1994: 105).

Teachers strongly affirmed that the changes in education policy and legislation made the commitment to inclusive education more difficult to maintain. The intensification and mechanization of the teaching act often led teachers to view inclusive priorities as an additional burden.

Teachers' often unmanageable workload led them to perceive children with special educational needs as being of 'second priority' for them while being the first priority of 'support' teachers. This practice reinforced the division between 'mainstream' and 'special' teachers; such allocation meant that mainstream teachers could present a façade of being supportive while taking the minimum responsibility for educating these children. In addition it perpetuated and even strengthened definitions of integration as being about 'specialism' and 'special teachers'.

In this context the increasing demand for the school to have sufficient resources to meet all of the expected goals strengthened the perception that integration was about 'resources'. This was understandable, considering that little had been restructured to fit the demands of teaching children with special educational needs while at the same time more and more had been added to the already existing structures and responsibilities of teachers' jobs. But such a preoccupation limited teachers' vision of integration and discouraged attempts to focus on the pedagogic aspects of the curriculum necessary for the inclusion of disabled children.

Children with special educational needs were in danger of experiencing a higher degree of exclusion within ordinary classrooms because of the mechanization of the teaching act, which reinforced a restrictive notion of learning, a specific image of children and a linear process of development. While political rhetoric talks about 'entitlement' in a broad and balanced curriculum, teachers talk about stronger external pressures to 'fit children in a specific system'. Teachers' struggles to avoid doing so represented their opposition to such political directives.

But all these elements, compounded with the intensification of competitiveness as an aim of education, were in contradiction with commitments to inclusive priorities. Under these conditions teachers were sceptical as to whether ordinary schools were the places in which children with special educational needs could be educated adequately.

Too many givens influenced and restricted definitions of integration. In turn, definitions of what constitutes 'resource children' were indicative of the way 'handicapped' identities are socially constructed. Such definitions were based on a number of institutional and practical restrictions. These included the cultural categories that teachers brought into their interactions with children with special educational needs (see Chapter 4). Definitions of the 'integrated resource' were contingent upon what the school could or could not offer. While teachers were aware of this, they tended to focus strongly on the within-the-child difficulties in justifying not only their attitudes towards integration but also the quality and the nature of education provided for children. Too many aspects of integration relied on children's perceived attributes even though such attributes were contingent on concerns, purposes, demands and pressures

emanating more from the school and classroom life than the children themselves. Further, a medical approach towards notions of disability had strengthened teachers' tendency to focus on different parts of the child (i.e. behavioural
and cognitive aspects) in justifying certain educational practices. Beyond this
approach, however, their tendency to focus strongly on within-the-child difficulties was both directly influenced by and influential upon two of the major
sub-roles of being a teacher: the disciplinarian and the instructor. Teachers' personal and professional achievement (their appreciation of the self as 'being
good at the job') was to be judged by the degree to which they could satisfac-
torily accomplish these sub-roles in their classrooms. This, in turn, was connected with being able to 'survive' within the classroom. Thus integration was
about conformity and discipline: often support teachers were called upon to
withdraw potentially 'disruptive' children from the class or to deal with them
in such a way as to ensure the smooth functioning of the ordinary system.

In institutions such as schools where conformity is a great, if not a central
institutional element, the process of integration was perceived as one of normalization. But the way normalization was both perceived and implemented
constituted just one more form of oppressive attitudes and practices towards
disabled children. The process of normalization in its applied form imposed a
negative connotation on 'difference'; its everyday practices were based on
modifying or tolerating difference. In addition the process of normalization
involves the cultural/ideological assumption that there exists an essential
homogeneity of cultural norms and values that individuals can adopt so as to
be ascribed a valued image and a culturally valued life (see Chapell 1994). All
the above reinforce the process of assimilation and the need for conformity,
rendering inclusive principles and practices difficult to implement.

However, teachers' positive attitudes towards the process of integration
originated from a recognition that integration was the best way to overcome
prejudices. They felt a moral responsibility to contribute to a positive epochal
shift, to a more caring – not necessarily inclusive – culture. They placed a great
emphasis on the social aspect of integration, often at the expense of the academic benefits for disabled children.

But the exploration of what 'social integration' involves suggests that the
issue of inclusion is much more complicated, and extends beyond school
boundaries. Indeed, it touches on the formation of self, and the ideologies and
values to be found in wider societal culture. Nowhere was this reflected more
than in the discussions I had with the children. Discussions with children can
reveal important messages about the nature of society in which we live. It is
through these discussions that one can realize that what are predominantly
viewed as natural and neutral occurrences are in fact socially created ideologies, history congealed into habit. Further, by observing and listening carefully to children I came to appreciate some aspects of children's culture. The
magnitude and multiplicities of their dimensions of power (both overt and
covert), and the complex intentions involved in their forming interpersonal
relationships (see Quicke and Winter 1994) go far beyond our efforts to capture reality in textual forms.

Social integration: culture and identity

While the dominant tendency in society has been to focus on the actual difficulties that disabled children might face in forming relationships, an exploration of children's attitudes towards their peers with Down's Syndrome
necessitates an exploration of the assumptions and values they hold, both on
issues of appearance and issues of mental disability. In interpersonal relationships between disabled and non-disabled children the former have to deal not
only with the actual difficulties originating out of a particular impairment but
also from the perceived restrictions associated with the cultural meanings
attributed to disabled children by their non-disabled peers. The opportunities
of different children with Down's Syndrome have been restricted and their
difficulties exacerbated, both because of the way mentally disabled children
have been regarded and treated and also because of the inaccurate stereotypes
which have been attached to their distinctive appearances. These assumptions
and stereotypes have been conceived by others previously and independently
from actual relationships with people with Down's Syndrome. Often these
individuals are rejected on the basis of their appearance rather than their
capabilities. The corporeal inscription of a disability such as Down's Syndrome
is just too much for pupils to ignore. In this case and as Marks (1994: 77) suggests, 'To be inscribed as physically different is to be conspicuous, and enlight-
ened educational and social policies appear to have done little to transform
that.'

Appearance in general is important because it is linked with cultural values
and assumptions that might not have any foundation in reality. However,
appearance in the context of disability is centrally important because it has
been used by non-disabled people as a social indication differentiating the
'normal' from the 'not normal'. It is the first challenge to what has been perceived as the 'social order of normalcy'. Simultaneously, this differentiation
serves the purpose of confirming that 'we' belong to the unstigmatized, creating in this way a particular group identity for the ones who have been perceived as different.

An important implication of this finding is that any attempt to change children's attitudes towards their disabled peers, in this case towards children
with Down's Syndrome, requires a change of attitudes towards what constitutes normalcy. This is because the two sets of attitudes are strongly connected, so that a change in one set should take into consideration a change in
the other. But we learn to place attitudes to normalcy at the very centre of our
lives, as children's emerging ideologies indicate. Here lies one of the multiple
reasons why particular negative attitudes towards disability, such as a strong
emphasis on a deficit approach to disabled people, are particularly resistant to
change.

The creation of more inclusive social practices requires that disability
awareness should extend further than the organization of the classroom
and/or the introduction of compartmentalized disability awareness programmes. It should be a cross-curriculum issue with an emphasis on reflecting

upon the values implicit in and transmitted through pedagogic practices. Schools' strong emphasis on conformity and normalization; the differentiation of pupils according to their intellectual competence and achievement: such values strengthen a particular notion of normalcy and are in contradiction with programmes that are applied in efforts to promote more inclusive relationships. Children should be encouraged to reflect on disability issues and to be critical of restricted notions of normalcy. Teachers' attitudes are of great importance because, as Chapter 5 illustrated, children's attitudes towards the process of integration reflected those of their teachers and/or wider society. Further, as Quicke *et al.* maintain,

> To many pupils . . . lessons about attitudes towards disability may seem paradoxical. On the one hand the teacher is encouraging critical engagement with ideas and practices which discriminate against persons with disabilities, whilst on the other the very same teacher may be identified with an authority which generates discriminatory attitudes of another kind.
> (Quicke *et al.* 1990: 128)

An additional reason for the complexities involved in changing children's attitudes towards their disabled peers is the linkage of specific attitudes with specific self-needs and priorities. The rules and sanctions of children's culture demand a high degree of conformity because acceptance is based very much on an instrumental notion of relationships. For instance, friendships are regarded as serving important self- rather than mutual interests. There is a continuous bargaining associated with efforts to 'control' the situation and to create a specific image and status necessary for the protection of self.

Simultaneously, within the realm of interactions children are learning the appropriate social order of behaviour contingent upon specific group contexts, structures and priorities. Deviations from what has been considered appropriate behaviour are perceived as threatening some of their primary interests-at-hand (see Chapter 6). The centrality of different interests varies, and it is this variation that influences how flexible and accepting different children or different groups are in their responses towards children who are perceived as exhibiting deviant behaviour. In this respect, it can be argued that within children's culture disability is regarded as a form of deviance, even though this issue is much more complicated as a process and needs further exploration (see Hargreaves *et al.* 1975). At this point, however, it is important to note that the perception that disabled children are deviant and the nature of the response towards behaviour exhibited by disabled peers is also influenced by the cultural meanings and categories that their peers bring into interactions with them.

Struggles for inclusive education: further considerations

Research such as this often seems to raise more questions than it answers. In fact, during the process of analysing, interpreting and discussing the findings, many issues emerged which were either beyond the scope of this study or for which there was a lack of adequate information and thus no safe interpretations could be made. There are, however, some areas/points of view that are particularly critical.

One of these issues, if we have any genuine concern to create a more inclusive society, is the need to approach attitudes towards integration from a different perspective. While notions of attitudes can be elusive, being influenced by a number of situational and personal variables, any attempt at attitudinal change should have as a starting point the realization that it is not solely the attributes of a disabled person and/or the nature of the disability that influence both teachers' and children's attitudes towards the process of integration. Attitudinal statements are highly linked with specific structures, values and ideologies that are to be found in the real world in which we all live. Thus any attempt to understand attitudes, and people's resistance to change, requires first and foremost that we understand the conflicts inherent in the reality within which attitudes are developed.

Currently conflicts and tensions concerning inclusive education have become more confusing and subtle. There is a plethora of contradicting ideologies and values; there is a babble of voices emerging out of the dynamics within which old assumptions no longer hold while new ideas and assumptions have not been internalized. To complicate issues further, critical terms either have no inherent meaning – certainly someone has to be appreciative of the multiple meanings already in existence – or they are used in different contexts serving different purposes.

Language is a significant tool in the struggle to define parts of the reality because communication itself has become a difficult and a confusing process – labels for social phenomena have lost their meaning because of the need to rethink and reconstruct certain terms and definitions. For instance, how are we to interpret notions such as 'democracy', 'equality', 'rights', 'choice' and 'professionalism' in a conservative highly technocratic and economically-led educational era? Such terms provide topics for interpretation, are themselves to be examined as interpretations, are subject to varying interpretations and can be examined – within this study's specific frame of reference – in terms of the extent to which they create structures that impinge upon the development of inclusive practices. Further, what does 'social policy' mean in a capitalist society and how do specific practices come to be defined and legitimized as 'social policies' even when they are not? These are critical questions and need further exploration if we are to understand 'the ways in which legislation and the vested interests of various professional groups may contribute to the legitimization of inequalities in the education of specific groups of children' (Vulliamy and Webb 1993: 189). They are also important in understanding why 'integration' is still surrounded by the same perennial questions (such as questions of resources, specialism, integration vs. segregation) as it was in the past when segregation was being justified.

I would not like to imply that the process of integration has been a static phenomenon – even though some facets of integration can demonstrate its stagnation as a process (see Marks 1994). Rather, the experience of conducting this study made me realize that the reasons for the resistance to changing certain attitudes – including policies and practices – are to be found elsewhere and not in the perceived abilities or 'disabilities' of disabled people. As Barton and Corbett (1993: 20) suggest, 'Our findings have supported the principle that there can be nothing simplistic about the process of change, which has to be both conceptual and structural.'

In this book it has been demonstrated that some objectives/definitions surrounding integration have in fact been consistent with extensive practices of segregation. Ideas arising from the philosophy and the practices of 'special' education have been imposed on the process of integration, limiting visions of inclusive practices. The language deployed and the ideologies underpinning it revealed that 'handicap', 'specialism' and notions of 'need' – despite the apparent implicit humanitarianism – were frequently-occurring themes surrounding what was to be perceived as being 'appropriate' within the social reality of schooling.

Inclusion is not about dumping children into already pressurized schools. In fact, inclusive policies and practices require that 'integration must be a policy, a programme, orientated towards its own destruction' (Brandson and Miller 1989: 161). As Slee has suggested, inclusive education 'necessitates a reconsideration of the complex and potent cocktail of pedagogy, curriculum, school organization and the ideologies that inform these components of schooling' (Slee 1993: 351). Inclusion is about the curriculum in its broader sense (see Wexler 1992; Apple 1993) and an exploration of the reasons that the educational apparatus has failed to create opportunities for all its learners regardless of their potential 'outcomes'. It is not about separated short-term programmes, special units, behaviouristic token-awarded approaches and experimental designs; it is about challenging issues of power, control, discipline, priorities and conformity to already established dominant sets of values.

Further, as Fulcher (1989a) has powerfully shown, it is not solely about laws. It is about commitment as well. Teachers play a significant role in the creation of more open and democratic structures. Teachers do not merely deliver the curriculum: they are the ultimate key to educational change and school improvement. 'Teacher expectations, sensitivities, priorities and values contribute to the quality of all pupils' learning experiences, and consequently teachers will influence what is taught, how it is taught, and the assessment of what has been taught' (Hartnett and Naish 1993: 341). Thus the creation of inclusive practices requires commitment on their part. However, it would be both naive and unfair to teachers to suggest that the creation of inclusive education can be based solely on their commitment. Given the multiple changes within schools and the contradictory pressures teachers have to assimilate, what they think about such factors and how they see their role changing are important topics of educational research. Discussions about teacher perceptions demand first of all an understanding of the context and work culture of schools. The importance of support, staff development and adequate resources are crucial issues to be tackled seriously. How do teachers view the changes imposed on them? What forms of opposition are they developing? What are the means they use in balancing their own ideologies with the ones they have to comply with? In what ways do they use already existing structures in pursuing their own interests-at-hand? These are questions which need to be examined further within specific school contexts to provide the sorts of support teachers are both entitled to and which are necessary in resisting idealized notions of change.

Furthermore, inclusive ideologies require changes at other levels of society as well. This includes the identification and exploration of the particular processes through which individuals are classified, objectified, individualized, disciplined, normalized and/or excluded from communities. In relation to integration, the medical and charitable/humanistic approaches towards disability and disabled people have contributed significantly to the fabrication of their inferior status by creating images that are connected with a particular notion of negatively valued difference (see Hewey 1992). This process has been further strengthened by the widespread dominance of values concerned with appearance, power and prestige, which in turn have been contingent on what seem to be the most valued elements of our existing society: competence, functionalism and commercial productivity.

In a society which is increasingly based on an ethic which gives emphasis to self-sufficiency, independence, status, success, power and wealth, desirable social features such as help, care and even interdependence have been used as indicators for legitimizing oppression, inferiority, marginalization and exclusion. Thus 'despite decades of progressive rhetoric . . . it is still the case that this minority group [the 'disabled'] feel stigmatized and boxed into stereotyped passive roles' (Quicke 1988: 167).

Because the struggle to challenge these sets of dominant values that oppress people as human beings is complex, difficult, brings discomfort and even is regarded in some circles as an 'unfashionable morality', the focus has been towards normalizing individuals who deviate from the norm in any respect by 'treating' and/or 'curing' their difference. Paradoxically, normalization is demanded in a world full of difference.

However, 'individuals may resist or contest the way they are constructed either by policy documents or by dominant cultural perspectives, and actively choose to construct their own subjectivities as other than compliant and conservative' (Marks 1994: 73). The way disabled pupils who are educated into ordinary schools construct views of their own subjectivities is a crucial issue and has not yet been seriously examined, thus restricting opportunities for expression. Disabled pupils' voices can enable us to understand that the way disabled children have traditionally been regarded reflects the philosophies and the policies of the relevant educational systems. Such accounts can help to show that specific images/identities of disabled children are social creations: the identities disabled individuals have created for themselves are different to the one imposed on them by official and/or educational systems.

Having said that, it would be a mistake to ignore that there are social relationships in which individual differences, irrespective of their degree and nature, are not only accepted but also celebrated. It could not be otherwise in a society that ascribes multiple meanings to cultural/social symbols. If that is not the case, how else are we able to interpret social relations in which persons defined by some as being 'severely and multiply handicapped' have been loved and befriended by others. Thus while it has been strongly emphasized that a sociology of exclusion is a serious and urgent task, we need a sociology of inclusion and acceptance as well. A sociology of acceptance should not replace the sociology of exclusion; rather, it can enlarge our understanding of relationships and would enable us to focus not only on 'what not to do' but how differences can be accepted and celebrated (see Bogdan and Taylor 1987). Further, the above suggestions are based on the assumption that it is the expression of individual subjectivities, especially by people who have been historically oppressed, that can help us understand the seriousness and importance of the questions they raise. Or, as Coleridge (1993: 36) puts it, 'Discrimination and prejudice create the sense of being disabled that leads to further discrimination and prejudice. How can this vicious circle be broken?'

In conclusion, I hope this book contributes to the encouragement of debate, although I am aware that it is just a small contribution to the framework rather than the answer to the problematics involved. I have tried to suggest further areas for investigation and to open up a wide range of questions. The endeavour to recognize the degree and nature of the disabling barriers to be overcome in the creation of more inclusive societies has no end. It can itself serve as the basis for change.

While knowledge remains partial and the demand for change continual, such change – towards a more inclusive society – requires us constantly to challenge inequalities of power, recognize the pre-eminent voice of the oppressed, and affirm who are the real knowers in this context: disabled people.

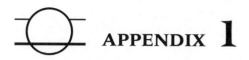 APPENDIX 1

The problem of ethical integrity

If we agree that the researcher is a human being as well, everyone has a limit to what s/he allows to happen in front of her eyes without intervening. In his article 'The problem of ethical integrity in participant observation', Jarvie (1982) explores the question of the relation between taking the role of stranger and that of a friend. He suggests that 'The unresolved identity crisis precipitates an integrity crisis and only by allowing one role to override the other, can the two crises be resolved' (p. 68). His examples are taken mainly from anthropological experiences and his analyses of idea versus practice in participant observation. All express the fieldworker's struggle both to be honest, fair and truthful, and to be an explorer. The conclusion he reached became a basic principle of this study:

> The observer does himself [*sic*] no harm if he [*sic*] acts in integrity towards his [*sic*] society and its values as far as possible. There is no reason to think the host people will not respect him [*sic*] more for this than for attempting to curry favour by pretending to go along with things that in truth offend, horrify or disgust him [*sic*]. Deception and hypocrisy are difficult enough to defend in the name of science. If we think science is served by entering into a full and equal relationship with the subjects of study, then both human and scientific integrity require that we do not artificially exclude from those relationships the tensions and clashes which enrich normal relationships. By and large anthropologists – I will add participant observers – act on this, but they do not give it due credit in their methodological discussions.
>
> (Jarvie 1982: 72)

Human and scientific integrity can eliminate the conflict that arises for the fieldworker from the internal pressure to be involved and the external pressure to be detached so as not to alter the environment she is studying – in other words 'to feel part of the group in his [*sic*] own marginal way' (Gans 1982: 55).

However, there is another and quite more problematic dilemma – involving conflict – that stems from the integrity of attachment to or detachment from the different interest-groups involved in the study. It is the ideological identification with the positions and the concerns of the different groups. To claim that at different times throughout the course of the entire research I did not 'take sides' by identifying myself and developing empathy for different groups would be a lie. I have worked as a teacher, and my professional experience sometimes meant that I prioritized teachers' concerns and constraints, as well as their 'interests-at-hand'. Consequently, perhaps I toned down my passion and idealism in regard to students' or parents' needs. At other times, having been a student for almost 25 years now, I could not help but identify with the pupils and the reality they have constructed within adults' institutionalized contexts. Taking the pupils' side made me feel angry towards educationists who try to mould and even modify pupils' actions and ways of thinking in the name of personal and social development.

A further source of conflict was my overt position about issues of disability and the way educational and other social and political apparatuses approach this issue. My involvement with disabled children and adults, and the opportunities I had to read or listen to their views, increased my desire and enthusiasm for further action. Often, however, my enthusiasm jarred with everyday exclusive processes and structures.

To summarize, I felt attached to groups which hold different hierarchical and social positions as well as needs and priorities that could not necessarily coincide. At the same time, though, I could not claim that I belonged to any of these groups because my position was somehow different from theirs. It is one thing to talk and empathize with a situation and another to actually experience it. It took a long time and it is still difficult, even now – to achieve a position of ideological integrity.

However, this kind of conflicting ideological attachment and detachment allowed me to experience internally similar conflicts between different groups when they endeavour to pursue their interests. Setting these conflicts in a wider perspective, perhaps they represent aspects of culture, if we view culture as 'an ongoing political struggle around the meaning given to actions of people located within unbounded asymmetrical power relationships' (LeCompte *et al.* 1992: 483).

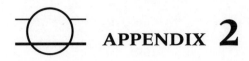 **APPENDIX 2**

Participants in the study

Teachers

| | Ordinary teachers | | | | Support teachers | | |
	Infants		Juniors		Infants		Juniors
Male	Female	Male	Female	Male	Female	Male	Female
0	4	4	2	1	3	2	3

Children

| | Children | |
	Male	Female
Years 1 and 2	14	15
Years 3 and 4	16	11
Years 3 and 4	16	14
Years 5 and 6	6	11

Total number of children: 103
Age range: 5 years 10 months to 11 years 6 months

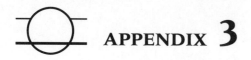 APPENDIX **3**

The role of the photograph in
interviews with the children

In the initial phase of the study one of the main concerns was the difficulty of discussing or trying to explore with children their images of and definitions about interactions with disabled children. There were two problems in particular: first, how to provide children with the opportunity to express the way they understood their realities without an adult's impositions; second, how to initiate discussions about their actual relationships with their peers with Down's Syndrome. My anxiety and ethical dilemma was that allowing children to talk about how they perceived their actual disabled peers might lead to an increased sense of judgement or scrutiny, with negative effects on their relationships.

Regarding the first question, I realized that it would be useful to orientate the discussion along broad open topics, allowing the children free rein to express their points of view. In other words I had in mind what Ann Lewis said when she reflected on her experience of interviewing children:

> They [children] were prompting one another with reference to things not known to the interviewer and this enabled individual children to amplify their responses . . . Their effectiveness may reflect the absence of the sorts of features (such as highly specific questions, and questions rather than comments) which diminish the quality and quantity of children's talk in conversation with adults.
>
> (Lewis 1992: 415)

This type of conversation demanded flexibility, from the researcher and also the ability to bring the discussion back on focus when the children got carried away on other irrelevant issues. It took me more than eight group discussions to feel comfortable with doing this. These initial group discussions enabled me not only to improve my skills on asking questions and listening, they also served as a platform for working out different ways of starting discussions about interactions with disabled children.

I was searching for an approach that would look at the realm of relationships, a device the children would have to think about and express feelings and opinions drawn from their everyday experiences. It had to be something that would act as a stimulus for the expression of images and definitions about disabled people, without specifying certain children as 'targets'.

Eventually I hit upon the idea of using a photograph portraying two girls, one non-disabled (Claire), the other (Sam), with Down's Syndrome. Neither girl attended the school or was known to the children in any way. Group discussions subsequently proved to be a quite stimulating experience. Thirty-four group discussions took place, each comprised of three pupils who were friends (see Cowie and Rudduck 1988). Each group discussion lasted approximately three hours with some breaks in between. Group discussions provided the opportunity for the expression of individual thoughts and experiences, disagreements as well as consensus. Also children expressed sets of beliefs that emerge during childhood and originate from a wider social spectrum. They offered me the opportunity to enhance the validity of this study because they were not only *talking* about their interactions, they were actually interacting as well.

Furthermore, the introduction of the photograph meant that I personally began to look at pictures from a different perspective – their social functioning both outside and inside a research context. I was also surprised to find out how many images we construct, unconsciously, through visual means (see Taylor 1992). The analysis of the role of photographs seems to reveal mechanisms that lead us to the formation and internalization of individual needs, concepts, values and attitudes. They include questions of interpretation, meaning and communication (see Webster 1980; Berger and Mohr 1982). 'They encompass the social practices, institutions and norms of a culture, providing information and expression that cannot be separated from our interpretation of any image' (English 1981: 12–13). At the same time the images that photographs create are drawn from already existing ideological and cultural assumptions that create more than one 'true' conception and presentation of reality:

> Since pictures often contain a wealth of information it is not surprising that more than one true thing can be said on the basis of a single image. When this happens, it only means that we are asking different questions which deserve and get different answers.
>
> (Becker 1979: 106)

The creation of different general questions and the way we answer them is highly connected with our familial, social and cultural environment. This is exactly what I wanted to find out from the children when I showed the photograph to them. I tried to explore and understand what kind of information children select from the available data – the photograph – and the ways they interpret it. In other words, I wished to find out 'what questions the picture was answering to the children' (Becker 1979: 101). Thus the photograph was introduced in order to provide the opportunity for the pupils to ask their own questions and offer their own answers instead of only the researcher asking predetermined questions.

A further research rationale for using a photograph was the exploration of the starting point in children's initial encounters with disabled children. Initial encounters between disabled people and others do not start from a neutral point. As Thomas (1978: 8) claimed, 'The disabled person has to deal with definitions of himself [*sic*] and his [*sic*] disability previously and independently conceived by others'. The introduction of the photograph simulated an artificial initial encounter between the participant children and the disabled girl of the picture, so that predefinitions and preconceptions about a disabled person were revealed. However, basing my assumptions and conclusions *solely* on the expressed opinions of the children towards a snapshot can become quite misleading. Participants were called to express opinions and feelings about someone whom they had never encountered before in their everyday life. Reflecting on the transcripts of children's discussions, it became evident that they responded more negatively to a picture of a disabled person than to their actual peers with Down's Syndrome. One highly probably explanation is that the children came in contact with the people in the photograph only once. The first was the last time as well. What was missing from the encounter with the individuals in the picture was a second or further opportunity for 'an active search for confirmatory evidence' (Hargreaves 1972: 33). Perceiving people and making inferences about them is a continuous process in which a lot of changes take place from our initial assumptions. If that is the case, then the reactions of the observer of the photograph is his/her initial interactions and assumptions about the other – thus we cannot talk about a process, only a static initial encounter. Contextualizing and triangulating the responses, though, was valuable as a way of increasing the opportunities for approaching and understanding the messages children revealed. Thus as the discussion progressed there was a 'natural' transition from hypothetical-fictional interactions to more concrete daily-based social encounters from children's own real world. In addition, over a period of more than one-and-a-half years, participant observations inside and outside of the class, as well as informal discussions with the children and their teachers, offered a number of opportunities for exploring how things were – or why they had been perceived by the participants – to be as they were and how things should be.

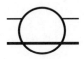

References

Abberley, P. (1987) The concept of oppression and the development of a social theory of disability, *Disability, Handicap and Society,* 2(1): 5–19.

Abberley, P. (1989) Disabled people, normality and social work, in L. Barton (ed.) *Disability and Dependency*. Lewes: The Falmer Press.

Abberley, P. (1992) Counting us out: a discussion of the OPCS disability surveys, *Disability, Handicap and Society*, 7(2): 139–56.

Abbot, D. and Croll, P. (1991) *Whole School Change under ERA*. Bristol: Redland Centre for Primary Education, Bristol Polytechnic. Presented at AERA, Chicago (April).

Ajzen, I. and Fishbein, M. (1977) Attitude-behaviour relations: a theoretical analysis and review of empirical research, *Psychological Research*, 84: 888–918.

Alexander, R., Rose, J. and Woodhead, C. (1993) The quality of teaching in primary schools, in R. Gomm and P. Woods (eds) *Educational Research in Action*, Vol. 2. London: Paul Chapman Publishing in association with The Open University.

Aloia, G. F. and MacMillan, D. L. (1983) Influence of the EMR label on initial expectations of regular-classroom teachers, *American Journal of Mental Deficiency*, 88(3): 255–62.

Amabile, T. M. and Stubbs, M. L. (eds) (1982) *Psychological Research in the Classroom: Issues for Educators and Researchers*. New York: Pergamon Press.

Apple, M. (1979) *Ideology and Curriculum*. London: Routledge and Kegan Paul.

Apple, M. (1993) *Official Knowledge: Democratic Education in a Conservative Age*. London: Routledge.

Argyle, M. (1975) *Bodily Communication*. London: Methuen.

Armistead, N. (1974) *Reconstructing Social Psychology*. Harmondsworth: Penguin.

Aspis, S. (1992) Integration, *Disability, Handicap and Society*, 7(3): 281–3.

Atkin, K. (1991) Health, illness, disability and Black minorities: a speculative critique of present day discourse, *Disability, Handicap and Society*, 6(1): 37–48.

Atkinson, P. (1992) *Understanding Ethnographic Texts*. Qualitative Research Methods Series, Vol. 25. London: Sage.

Bak, J. J. and Siperstein, J. N. (1986) Protective effects of the label 'mentally retarded' on children's attitudes towards mentally retarded peers, *American Journal of Mental Deficiency*, 91(1): 95–7.

Baker, J. L. and Gottlieb, J. (1980) Attitudes of teachers toward mainstreaming retarded children, in J. Gottlieb (ed.) *Education of Mentally Retarded Persons in the Mainstream*. Baltimore, MD: University Park Press.

Baldwin, W. K. (1958) The exceptional position of mentally handicapped children in the regular classes in the public school, *Exceptional Children*, 25: 106–8.

Ball, S. J. (1984) Banding, identity and experience, in M. Hammersley and P. Woods (eds) *Life in School: The Sociology of Pupil Culture*. Milton Keynes: Open University Press.

Ball, S. J. (1994) *Education Reform: A Critical and Post-Structural Approach*. Buckingham: Open University Press.

Ball, S. J., Bowe, R. and Gewirtz, C. (1994) Market forces and parental choice: self-interest and competitive advantage in education, in S. Tomlinson (ed.) *Educational Reform and its Consequences*. London: IPPR/Rivers Oram Press.

Barnett, D. and Zucker, K. (1980) The others concept: explorations into the quality of children's interpersonal relationships, in H. Foot, A. Chapman and J. Smith (eds) *Friendship and Social Relations in Children*. New York: John Wiley and Sons.

Barton, L. (1986) The politics of special educational needs, *Disability, Handicap and Society*, 1(3): 273–89.

Barton, L. (1987) Keep schools in line, in T. Booth and D. Coulby (eds) *Producing and Reducing Disaffection: Curricula for All*. Milton Keynes: Open University Press.

Barton, L. (ed.) (1988) *The Politics of Special Educational Needs*, Disability, Handicap and Life Chances Series. Lewes: The Falmer Press.

Barton, L. (ed.) (1989) *Disability and Dependency*. Lewes: The Falmer Press.

Barton, L. (1991) Disability: the necessity of a socio-political perspective. Conference paper presented at the International Conference in Oakland, California (June).

Barton, L. (1995) The politics of education for all. Paper presented at the International Special Education Congress in Birmingham (10–13 April).

Barton, L. and Corbett, J. (1993) Special needs in further education: the challenge of inclusive provision, *European Journal of Special Needs Education*, 8(1): 14–23.

Barton, L. and Meighan, R. (eds) (1979) *Schools, Pupils and Deviance*. England: Nafferton Books.

Barton, L. and Oliver, M. (1992) Special needs: a personal trouble or public issue? in M. Arnot and L. Barton (eds) *Voicing Concerns: Sociological Perspectives on Contemporary Education Reforms*. Oxford: Triangle Books.

Barton, L. and Tomlinson, S. (eds) (1984) *Special Education and Social Interest*, Croom Helm Series on Special Educational Needs: Policy, Practices and Social Issues. London: Croom Helm.

Barton, L. and Walker, S. (eds) (1981) *Schools, Teachers and Teaching*. Lewes: The Falmer Press.

Bates, I. and Rowland, S. (1988) Is student-centred pedagogy 'progressive' educational practice? *Journal of Further and Higher Education*, 12(3): 5–20.

Becker, H. (1979) Do photographs tell the truth? in D. T. Cook and S. C. Reichardt (eds) *Qualitative and Quantitative Methods in Evaluation Research*. London: Sage.

Becker, H. S. and Geer, B. (1982) Participant observation: the analysis of qualitative field data, in R. G. Burgess (ed.) *Field Research: A Sourcebook and Field Manual*. London: Allen and Unwin.

Bell, R. (1981) *Worlds of Friendship*. London: Sage.

Bentler, P. M. and Speckart, G. (1979) Models of attitude-behavior relations, *Psychological Review*, 86(5): 452–64.

Bentler, P. M. and Speckart, G. (1981) Attitudes 'cause' behaviors: a structural equation analysis, *Journal of Personality and Social Psychology*, 40: 226–38.

Berger, J. and Mohr, J. (1976) *A Fortunate Man*. London: Writers and Readers.

Berger, J. and Mohr, J. (1982) *Another Way of Telling*. London: Writers and Readers.

Berlak, A. and Berlak, H. (1981) *Dilemmas of Schooling: Teaching and Social Change*. London: Methuen.

Besag, V. (1989) *Bullies and Victims in Schools*. Milton Keynes: Open University Press.

Bines, H. (1995) Risk, routine and reward: confronting personal and social constructs in research on special educational needs, in P. Clough and L. Barton (eds) *Making Difficulties: Research and the Construction of SEN*. London: Paul Chapman Publishing.

Black, P. (1994) Alternative education policies: assessment and testing, in S. Tomlinson (ed.) *Educational Reform Act and its Consequences*. London: IPPR/Rivers Oram Press.

Blishen, E. (ed.) (1969) *The School that I'd Like*. Harmondsworth: Penguin Books.

Blyth, A. (1990) Social demands and schools' responses, in N. Proctory (ed.) *The Aims of Primary Education and the National Curriculum*. Lewes: The Falmer Press.

Bogdan, R. G. and Taylor, S. (1987) Toward a sociology of acceptance: the other side of the study of deviance, *Social Policy*, Fall: 34–9.

Bolton, E. (1994) Alternative education policies: school inspection, in S. Tomlinson (ed.) *Educational Reform Act and its Consequences*. London: IPPR/Rivers Oram Press.

Booth, T. (1981) Demystifying integration, in W. Swann (ed.) *The Practice of Special Education*. Oxford: Blackwell.

Booth, T. (1983) Policies towards the integration of mentally handicapped children in education, *Oxford Review of Education*, 9(3): 255–68.

Booth, T. (1985) Labels and their consequences, in D. Lane and B. Stratford (eds) *Current Approaches to Down's Syndrome*. London: Holt, Rinehart and Winston.

Booth, T. and Statham, J. (1982) *Parent's Choice, Establishing a Unit for Children with Down's Syndrome in an Ordinary School*. London: Campaign for Mentally Handicapped People.

Borsay, A. (1986) Personal trouble or public issue? Towards a model of policy for people with physical and mental disabilities, *Disability, Handicap and Society*, 1(2): 179–95.

Bowman, I. (1989) Teacher training and the integration of handicapped pupils: a Unesco study, in N. Jones (ed.) *Special Educational Needs Review*, 1. London: The Falmer Press.

Branson, J. and Miller, D. (1989) Beyond integration policy – the deconstruction of disability, in L. Barton (ed.) *Integration: Myth or Reality?* Lewes: The Falmer Press.

Brehony, K. J. (1990) Neither rhyme nor reason: primary schooling and the National Curriculum, in M. Flude and M. Hammer (eds) *The Education Reform Act 1988: Its Origins and Implications*. Lewes: The Falmer Press.

Brisenden, S. (1986) Independent living and the medical model of disability, *Disability, Handicap and Society*, 1(2): 173–8.

Bromfield, R., Wiz, J. R. and Messer, T. (1986) Children's judgments and attributions in response to the mentally retarded label: a developmental approach, *Journal of Abnormal Psychology*, 95: 81–7.

Buckley, S. (1985) Attaining basic skills: reading, writing and number, in D. Lane and B. Stratford (eds) *Current Approaches to Down's Syndrome*. London: Holt, Rinehart and Winston.

Burgess, R. G. (1981) Keeping a research diary, *Journal of Education*, 11(1): 75–81.

Burgess, R. G. (ed.) (1982) *Field Research: A Source Book and Field Manual*. London: Allen and Unwin.

Burgess, R. G. (1984) *In the Field*. London: Allen and Unwin.

Burgess, R. G. (ed.) (1985) *Field Methods in the Study of Education*. Lewes: The Falmer Press.

Cameron, K. C. and Whetten, D. A. (eds) (1983) *Organizational Effectiveness: A Comparison of Multiple Models*. New York: Academic Press.

Campaign for Mentally Handicapped People (1982) *Parents' Choice: Establishing a Unit for Children with Down's Syndrome in an Ordinary School*. London: CHM.

Campbell, R. J., Evans, L. and Neil, S. R. (1993) The use and management of infant teachers' time: some policy issues. *Warwick Papers on Education Policy*, No. 3. Stoke-on-Trent: Trentham Books.

Candappa, M. and Burgess, R. (1989) 'I'm not handicapped – I'm different': normalization, hospital care and mental handicap, in L. Barton (ed.) *Disability and Dependency*. Lewes: The Falmer Press.

Carr, W. and Quicke, J. (1990) An impossible dream? Comprehensive principles and the politics of inequality in British education, *Revista Española de Pedagogia*, 187: 429–40.

Carrier, J. G. (1990) Special education and the explanation of pupil performance, *Disability, Handicap and Society*, 5(3): 211–25.

Carroll, A. (1967) The effects of segregated and partially integrated school programs on self-concept and academic achievement of educable mentally retarded, *Exceptional Children*, 34: 93–6.

Carter, D. E., Carter, L. D. and Benson, F. W. (1980) Interracial acceptance in the classroom, in H. C. Foot, A. J. Chapman and J. R. Smith (eds) *Friendship and Social Relations in Children*. Chichester: John Wiley and Sons.

Cassidy, V. M. and Stanton, J. E. (1959) *An Investigation of Factors Involved in the Educational Placement of Mentally Retarded Children*. Columbus: Ohio State University.

Cavallaro, S. A. and Porter, R. H. (1980) Peer preferences of at risk and normally developing children in a pre-school mainstream classroom, *American Journal of Mental Deficiency*, 84(4): 357–66.

Chapell, A. L. (1994) A question of friendship: community care and the relationships of people with learning difficulties, *Disability and Society*, 9(4): 419–34.

Clough, P. (1995) Problems of identity and method in the investigation of special educational needs, in P. Clough and L. Barton (eds) *Making Difficulties: Research and the Construction of SEN*. London: Paul Chapman Publishing.

Clough, P. and Lindsay, G. (1991) *Integration and the Support Service: Changing Roles in Special Education*. Windsor: NFER-Nelson.

Cohen, L. and Mannion, L. (1980) *Research Methods in Education*. London: Croom Helm.

Cohen, S. and Taylor, L. (1976) *Escape Attempts: The Theory and Practice of Resistance to Everyday Life*. London: Pelican Books.

Coleridge, P. (1993) *Disability, Liberation, and Development*. Oxford: Oxfam Publications.

Collins, J. (1994) 'The silent minority: developing talk in the primary classroom', unpublished Ph.D. thesis. University of Sheffield.

Corbett, J. (1991) So, who wants to be normal? *Disability, Handicap and Society*, 6(3): 259–60.

Cowie, H. and Rudduck, J. (1988) *Co-operative Group Work: An Overview. Learning Together – Working Together*, Vol. 1. London: BP Educational Service.

Croll, P. and Moses, D. (1985) *One in Five: The Assessment and Incidence of Special Educational Needs, Systematic Classroom Observation*. London: Routledge and Kegan Paul.

Dandy, J. and Callen, C. (1988) Integration and mainstreaming: a review of the efficacy of mainstreaming and integration for mentally handicapped pupils, *Educational Psychology*, 8(3): 332–41.

Davidson, I., Woodill, G. and Bredberg, E. (1994) Images of disability in 19th century British children's literature, *Disability and Society*, 9(1): 33–46.

Davies, B. (1982) *Life in the Classroom and Playground: The Accounts of Primary School Children*. London: Routledge and Kegan Paul.

Davies, B. (1989) *Frogs and Snails and Feminist Tales: Preschool Children and Gender*. Sydney: Allen and Unwin.

Dearing, D. (1994) *The National Curriculum and its Assessment: Final Report*. London: SEAC.

Delamont, S. (1992) *Fieldwork in Educational Settings: Methods, Pitfalls and Perspectives*. Lewes: The Falmer Press.

Delamont, S. and Galton, M. (1986) *Inside the Secondary Classroom*. London: Routledge and Kegan Paul.

Delamont, S. and Hamilton, D. (1986) Revisiting classroom research: a continuing cautionary tale, in M. Hammersley (ed.) *Controversies in Classroom Research*. Milton Keynes: Open University Press.

Department of Education and Science (1987a) *Grant Maintained Schools: Consultation Papers*. London: DES.

Department of Education and Science (1987b) *The National Curriculum 5–6: A Consultation Document*. London: DES.

Dunn, K. (1991) 'Working class culture and co-operation: a case study of schooling and social life in a Yorkshire mining community', unpublished Ph.D. thesis. University of Sheffield.

Easterday, L., Papademas, D., Schorr, L. and Valentine, C. (1982) The making of a female researcher: role problems in fieldwork, in R. G. Burgess (ed.) *Field Research: A Sourcebook and Field Manual*. London: Allen and Unwin.

Eayrs, C., Ellis, N. and Jones, R. (1993) Which label? An investigation into the effects of terminology on public perceptions of and attitudes towards people with learning difficulties, *Disability, Handicap and Society*, 8(2): 111–28.

Edgerton, R. B. (1967) *The Cloak of Competence: Stigma in the Lives of the Mentally Retarded*. Berkeley: University of California Press.

Elliot, N. (1990) The life of childhood: environment and experience, in N. Proctor (ed.) *The Aims of Primary Education and the National Curriculum*. Lewes: The Falmer Press.

English, E. D. (1981) *Political Uses of Photography in the Third French Republic 1871–1914*. Ann Arbor, MI: UMI Research Press.

Evans, J., Goacher, B., Wedell, K. and Welton, J. (1990) The implementation of the 1981 Education Act, in N. Jones (ed.) *Special Educational Needs Review*, Vol. 3. Lewes: The Falmer Press.

Feldman, D. and Altman, R. (1985) Conceptual systems and teacher attitudes toward regular classroom placement of mildly mentally retarded students, *American Journal of Mental Deficiency*, 89(4): 345–51.

Finkelstein, V. (1980) *Attitudes and Disabled People*. New York: Work Rehabilitation Fund.

Firth, H. and Rapley, M. (1990) *From Acquaintance to Friendship: Issues for People with Learning Disabilities*. Birmingham: BIMH Publications.

Fishbein, M. and Ajzen, I. (1974) Attitudes toward objects as predictors of single and multiple behavioral criteria, *Psychological Review*, 81: 59–74.

Fishbein, M. and Ajzen, M. (1975) *Belief, Attitude, Intention and Behaviour: An Introduction to Theory and Research*. Reading, MA: Addison-Wesley.

Foot, H., Chapman, A. and Smith, J. (eds) (1980) *Friendship and Social Relations in Children*. New York: John Wiley and Sons.

Frankenberg, R. (1982) Participant observers, in R. G. Burgess (ed.) *Field Research: A Sourcebook and Field Manual*. London: Allen and Unwin.

Freire, P. (1985) *The Politics of Education: Culture, Power and Liberation*. London: Macmillan.

Freilich, M. (ed.) (1977) *Marginal Natives at Work: Anthropologists in the Field*. New York: Wiley.

French, S. (1993) Disability, impairment or something in between? in J. Swain, V. Finkelstein, S. French and M. Oliver (eds) *Disabling Barriers – Enabling Environments*. London: Sage in association with The Open University.

Fulcher, G. (1989a) *Disabling Policies? A Comparative Approach to Education Policy and Disability*, Disability, Handicap and Life Chances Series. Lewes: The Falmer Press.

Fulcher, G. (1989b) Disability: a social construction, in G. Lupton and J. Najman (eds) *Sociology of Health and Illness*. Victoria, Australia: Macmillan.

Fulcher, G. (1995) Excommunicating the severely disabled: struggles, policy and researching, in P. Clough and L. Barton (eds) *Making Difficulties: Research and the Construction of SEN*. London: Paul Chapman Publishing.

Furlong, V. (1976) Interaction sets in the classroom: towards a study of pupil knowledge, in M. Hammersley and P. Woods (eds) *The Process of Schooling*. London: Routledge and Kegan Paul in association with The Open University Press.

Galloway, D. and Goodwin, C. (1987) *Educating Slow Learning and Maladjusted Children: Integration or Segregation?* London: Longman.

Gans, H. J. (1982) The participant observer as a human being: observations on the personal aspects of fieldwork, in R. G. Burgess (ed.) *Field Research: A Sourcebook and Field Manual*. London: Allen and Unwin.

Ginsburg, M., Mayenn, R. and Miller, H. (1980) Teachers' conception of professionalism and trade unionism: an ideological analysis, in P. Woods (ed.) *Teacher Strategies*. London: Croom Helm.

Giroux, H. (1984) Ideology, agency and the process of schooling, in L. Barton and S. Walker (eds) *Social Crisis and Educational Research*. London: Croom Helm.

Goffman, E. (1961) *Encounters: Two Studies in the Sociology of Interaction*. Indianapolis, IN: Bobbs-Merrill.

Goffman, E. (1963) *Stigma: Notes on the Management of Spoiled Identity*. Englewood Cliffs, NJ: Prentice-Hall.

Goffman, E. (1971) *The Presentation of Self in Everyday Life*. Harmondsworth: Penguin Books.

Gold, D. (1994) We don't call it a 'circle': the ethos of a support group, *Disability and Society*, 9(4): 435–52.

Goode, D. A. (1984) Socially produced identities, intimacy and the problem of competence among the retarded, in L. Barton and S. Tomlinson (eds) *Special Education and Social Interests*. London: Croom Helm.

Goodman, H., Gottlieb, J. and Harrison, R. H. (1972) Social acceptance of EMRs integrated into a non-graded elementary school, *American Journal of Mental Deficiency*, 76(2): 412–17.

Gottlieb, J. (1974) Attitudes toward retarded children: effects of labelling and academic performance, *American Journal of Mental Deficiency*, 79(3): 268–73.

Gottlieb, J. (1986) Mainstreaming: fulfilling the promise? *American Journal of Mental Deficiency*, 86(2): 115–26.

Gottlieb, J. and Siperstein, G. (1976) Attitudes towards mentally retarded persons: effects of attitude referent specificity, *American Journal of Mental Deficiency*, 80(4): 376–81.

Guralnick, M. J. and Croom, J. M. (1980) Peer interactions in mainstreamed and specialized classrooms: a comparative analysis, *Exceptional Children*, 54: 415–25.

Hammersley, M. and Scarth, J. (1993) Beware of wise men bearing gifts: a case study in the misuse of educational research, in R. Gomm and P. Woods (eds) *Educational Research in Action*, Vol. 2. London: Paul Chapman Publishing in association with The Open University Press.

Hargreaves, A. (1993) Time and teachers' work: an analysis of the intensification thesis, in R. Gomm and P. Woods (eds) *Educational Research in Action*, Vol. 2. London: Paul Chapman Publishing in association with The Open University.

Hargreaves, A. (1994) *Changing Teachers, Changing Times: Teachers' Work and Culture in the Postmodern Age*. London: Cassell.

Hargreaves, D. H. (1967) *Social Relations in a Secondary Modern School*. London: Routledge and Kegan Paul.

Hargreaves, D. H. (1972) *Interpersonal Relations and Education*. London: Routledge and Kegan Paul.

Hargreaves, D. H. (1982) *The Challenge for the Comprehensive School: Culture, Curriculum and Community*. London: Routledge and Kegan Paul.

Hargreaves, D. H., Hester, S. K. and Mellor, F. J. (1975) *Deviance in Classrooms*. London: Routledge and Kegan Paul.

Harry (1991) Harry talks, *Zero Three*, 5: 10–12.

Hartnett, A. and Naish, M. (1993) Democracy, teachers and the struggles for education: an essay in the political economy of teacher education, *Curriculum Studies*, 1(3): 335–48.

Hegarty, S. (1987) *Meeting Special Needs in Ordinary Schools*. London: Cassell.

Hegarty, S. (1988) Past, current and future research on integration: an NFER perspective, in N. Jones (ed.) *Special Educational Needs Review*, Vol. 1. Lewes: The Falmer Press.

Hegarty, S. and Pocklington, K. (1981) *Educating Pupils with Special Educational Needs in the Ordinary School*. Windsor: NFER-Nelson.

Hellenbec, M. J. and McMaster, D. (1991) Disability simulation for regular education students, *Teaching Exceptional Children*, 23(3): 12–15.

Hercock, T. (1991) Children with special needs in mainstream schools, *Education Guardian*, 10 December.

Heritage, J. (1974) Assessing people, in N. Armistead (ed.) *Reconstructing Social Psychology*. Harmondsworth: Penguin.

Hewey, D. (1992) *The Creatures Time Forgot: Photography and Disability Imagery*. London: Routledge.

Hill, J. (1992) 'Special schooling, statementing procedures and gender: a sociological case-study analysis', unpublished Ph.D. thesis. School of Education: Sheffield City Polytechnic.

Hirst, P. and Woolley, P. (1982) *Social Relations and Human Attributes*. London: Tavistock.

Hoben, M. (1980) Toward integration in the mainstream, *Exceptional Children*, 47: 100–5.

Homans, G. C. (1951) *The Human Group*. London: Routledge and Kegan Paul.

Hunt, F. J. (1990) *The Social Dynamics of Schooling: Participants, Priorities and Strategies*. Lewes: The Falmer Press.

Jackson, P. W. (1968) *Life in Classrooms*. New York: Holt, Rinehart and Winston.

James, A. (1993) *Childhood Identities, Self and the Social Relationships in the Experience of the Child*. Edinburgh: Edinburgh University Press.

Jarvie, I. C. (1982) The problem of ethical integrity in participant observation, in R. G. Burgess (ed.) *Field Research: A Sourcebook and Field Manual*. London: Allen and Unwin.

Jenkins, J. R., Odom, L. S. and Speltz, M. L. (1989) Effects of social integration on pre-school children with handicaps, *Exceptional Children*, 55(5): 420–8.

Johnson, R. T. and Johnson, D. W. (1981) Building friendships between handicapped and non-handicapped students: effects of co-operative and individualistic instruction, *American Educational Research Journal*, 18(4): 415–23.

Jones, E. (1991) Concert addicts, *Zero Three*, 5: 7–9.

Jones, N. (1985) Extending the concept of normality, *Education*, 166: 24.

Jordan, A. M. (1959) Personal-social traits of mentally handicapped children, in T. G. Thurston (ed.) *An Evaluation of Educating Mentally Handicapped Children in Special Classes and in Regular Classes*. Chapel Hill: University of North Carolina, School of Education.

Jupp, K. (1992) *Everyone Belongs: Mainstream Education for Children with Severe Learning Difficulties*. London: Souvenir Press.

Kahle, L. R. (1984) *Attitudes and Social Adaptation: A Person–Situation Interact Approach*, International Series, Experimental Social Psychology, Vol. 8. New York: Pergamon Press.

Karagiannis, T. (1988) 'Attitudes towards integrating children with Down's Syndrome', unpublished master's thesis. McGill University, Montreal.

Keddie, N. (1971) Classroom knowledge, in M. Young (ed.) *Knowledge and Control*. London: Macmillan.

Kefala, E. (1991) In my view, *Zero Three*, 5: 19–20.

Kelly, A. V. (1990) *The National Curriculum: A Critical Review*. London: Paul Chapman Publishing.

Kennedy, A. B. and Thurman, S. K. (1982) Inclinations of non-handicapped children to help their handicapped peers, *The Journal of Special Education*, 16(3): 319–27.

Kurtz, P. D., Harrison, M., Neisworth, J. T. and Jones, R. T. (1977) Influence of 'mentally retarded' label on teachers' non-verbal behaviour toward pre-school children, *American Journal of Mental Deficiency*, 82: 204–6.

Kyle, C. and Davies, K. (1991) Attitudes of mainstream pupils towards mental retardation: pilot study at a Leeds secondary school, *British Journal of Special Education*, 18(3): 103–6.

LeCompte, M. D., Millray, W. L. and Preissle, J. (1992) *The Handbook of Qualitative Research in Education*. San Diego, CA: Academic Press.

Levinger, G. (1974) A three-level approach to attraction: towards an understanding of pair relatedness, in T. L. Huston (ed.) *Foundations of Interpersonal Attraction*. New York: Academic Press.

Lewis, A. (1992) Group child interviews as a research tool, *British Educational Research Journal*, 18(4): 413–21.

Lewis, A. and Lewis, V. (1988) Young children's attitudes after a period of integration towards peers with severe learning difficulties, *European Journal of Special Needs Education*, 3(3): 161–71.

Leyser, Y. and Abrams, P. D. (1983) A shift to the positive: an affective programme for changing pre-service teachers' attitudes towards the disabled, *Education Review*, 35(1): 36–43.

Likert, T. (1932) A technique for the measurement of attitude, *Archives of Psychology*, 140: 1–55.

Llewellyn, R. (1983) Future health services – a challenge for disabled people, *Australian Rehabilitation Review*, 7(4): 24–31.

Lortie, D. C. (1975) *Schoolteacher*. Chicago: University of Chicago Press.

Lynas, W. (1986) Pupils attitudes to integration, *British Journal of Special Education*, 13(1): 45–57.

Lynch, J. (1987) *Prejudice Reduction and the Schools*. London: Cassell.

MacMillan, D. L., Jones, R. L. and Aloia, G. F. (1974) The mentally retarded label: a theoretical analysis and review of research, *American Journal of Mental Deficiency*, 79: 241–61.

Marks, G. (1994) 'Armed now with hope . . .': the construction of the subjectivity of students within integration, *Disability and Society*, 9(1): 71–84.

Mayrowitz, J. H. (1962) Peer groups and special classes, *Mental Retardation*, 5: 23–6.

McGhee, P. and Chapman, A. (1980) *Children's Humour*. Chichester: John Wiley and Sons.

McHale, S. and Simeonsson, R. J. (1980) Effects of interaction on non-handicapped children's attitudes toward autistic children, *American Journal of Mental Deficiency*, 85: 18–24.

Mehan, H. (1993) 'Why I like to look': on the use of videotape as an instrument in educational research, in M. Schratz (ed.) *Qualitative Voices in Educational Research*. London: The Falmer Press.

Mehan, H., Hertweck, A. and Meihls, L. (1986) *Handicapping the Handicapped: Decision Making in Students' Educational Careers*. Stanford, CA: Stanford University Press.

Meighan, R. (1981) *A Sociology of Educating*. London: Holt, Rinehart and Winston.

Mercer, J. and Richardson, J. (1975) 'Mental retardation' as a social problem, in N. Hobbs (ed.) *Issues in the Classification of Children*, Vol. 11. San Francisco, CA: Jossey-Bass.

Miller, C. T. and Gibbs, E. D. (1984) High school students' attitudes and actions toward 'slow learners', *American Journal of Mental Deficiency*, 89(2): 156–66.

Mittler, P. (1992) Whose needs? Whose interests? in G. Fairbairn and S. Fairbairn (eds) *Integrating Special Children: Some Ethical Issues*. Aldershot: Avebury Ashgate Publishing.

Morris, J. (1992) Personal and political: a feminist perspective on researching physical disability, *Disability, Handicap and Society*, 7(2): 157–66.

Morss, J. R. (1985) Early cognitive development: difference or delay, in D. Lane and B. Stratford (eds) *Current Approaches to Down's Syndrome*. London: Holt, Rinehart and Winston.

Mousley, J., Rice, M. and Tregenza, K. (1993) Integration of students with disabilities into regular schools: policy in use, *Disability, Handicap and Society*, 8(1): 59–70.

Murphy, R. (1990) National assessment proposals: analysing the debate, in M. Flude and M. Hammer (eds) *The Education Reform Act 1988: Its Origins and Implication*. Lewes: The Falmer Press.

National Curriculum Council (1992) *The National Curriculum and Pupils with Severe Learning Difficulties*. York: NCC.

Nias, J. (1989) *Primary Teachers Talking*. London: Routledge.

O'Hear, P. (1994) An alternative national curriculum, in S. Tomlinson (ed.) *Educational Reform and its Consequences*. London: IPPR/Rivers Oram Press.

Oliver, M. (1985) The integration–segregation debate: some sociological considerations, *British Journal of Sociology of Education*, 6(1): 74–91.

Oliver, M. (1986) Social theory and disability: some theoretical issues, *Disability, Handicap and Society*, 1(1): 5–17.

Oliver, M. (1987) Redefining disability: a challenge to research, *Research in Special Needs*, 5(1): 12–24.

Oliver, M. (1992a) Changing the social relations of research production, *Disability, Handicap and Society*, 7(2): 101–14.

Oliver, M. (1992b) Intellectual masturbation: a rejoinder to Soder and Booth, *European Journal of Special Education*, 7(1): 20–8.

Opie, I. and Opie, P. (1959) *The Lore and Language of Schoolchildren*. Oxford: The Clarendon Press.

Perske, R. and Perske, M. (1988) *Circles of Friends: People with Disabilities and their Friends Enrich the Lives of One Another*. Nashville, TN: Abingdon Press.

Peters, S. (1995) Disability baggage: changing the educational research terrain, in P. Clough and L. Barton (eds) *Making Difficulties: Research and the Construction of SEN*. London: Paul Chapman Publishing.

Peterson, N. L. and Haralick, J. G. (1977) Integration of handicapped and non-handicapped pre-schoolers: an analysis of play behaviour, *Education and Training of the Mentally Retarded*, 1: 235–45.

Pinhas, A. G. and Schmelkin, L. P. (1989) Administrators and teachers' attitudes toward mainstreaming, *Remedial and Special Education*, 10(4): 38–43.

Pollard, A. (1985) *The Social World of the Primary School*. London: Holt, Rinehart and Winston.

Pollard, A. (1990) The aims of primary school teachers, in N. Proctor (ed.) *The Aims of Primary Education and the National Curriculum*. London: The Falmer Press.

Pollard, A. (1992) Teachers' responses to the reshaping of primary education, in M. Arnot and L. Barton (eds) *Voicing Concerns: Sociological Perspectives on Contemporary Education Reforms*. Wallingford: Triangle.

Pollard, A., Broadfoot, P., Croll, P., Osborn, M. and Abbott, D. (1994) *Changing English Primary Schools? The Impact of the Education Reform Act at Key Stage One*. London: Cassell.

Powell, M. and Solity, J. (1990) *Teachers in Control: Cracking the Code*. London: Routledge.

Quicke, J. C. (1981) Special educational needs and the comprehensive principle: some implications of ideological critique, *Remedial Education*, 16(2): 61–5.

Quicke, J. C. (1985) *Disability in Modern Children's Fiction*. London: Croom Helm.

Quicke, J. C. (1986) Pupil culture, peer tutoring and special educational needs, *Disability, Handicap and Society*, 1(2): 147–64.

Quicke, J. C. (1988) 'Speaking out': the political career of Hellen Keller, *Disability, Handicap and Society*, 3(2): 167–71.

Quicke, J. C. (1989) Mental handicap awareness and gender relations in a comprehensive school, in C. Roaf and H. Bines (eds) *Needs, Rights and Opportunities*. Lewes: The Falmer Press.

Quicke, J. C. (1991) Prejudice elimination as an educational aim, *British Journal of Educational Studies*, 39(1): 45–58.

Quicke, J. and Winter C. (1994) Education, co-operation and the cultural practices of assertive girls, *International Studies in Sociology of Education*, 4(2): 173–90.

Quicke, J., Beasley, K. and Morrison, C. (1990) *Challenging Prejudice through Education: The Story of a Mental Handicap Awareness Curriculum Project*. Lewes: The Falmer Press.

Reynolds, B. J., Reynolds, J. M. and Mark, F. D. (1982) Elementary teachers' attitudes toward mainstreaming educable mentally retarded students, *Education and Training of the Mentally Retarded*, 17(3): 171–6.

Rieser, R. and Mason, M. (1992) *Disability Equality in the Classroom: A Human Rights Issue*. London: Disability, Equality in Education.

Roaf, C. and Bines, H. (eds) (1989) *Needs, Rights and Opportunities: Developing Approaches to Special Education*. Lewes: The Falmer Press.

Roffey, S., Tarrant, T. and Majors, K. (1994) *Young Friends: Schools and Friendship*. London: Cassell.

Rogers, C. (1978) The child's perception of other people, in J. McGurk (ed.) *Issues in Childhood Social Development*. London: Methuen.

Roiser, M. (1974) Asking silly questions, in N. Armistead (ed.) *Reconstructing Social Psychology*. Harmondsworth: Penguin.

Rosen, M., Clark, G. and Kivitz, M. (eds) (1976) *The History of Mental Retardation: Collected Papers*. London: University Park Press.

Rosenthal, R. and Jacobson, L. (1968) *Pygmalion in the Classroom: Expectations and Pupils' Intellectual Development*. New York: Holt, Rinehart and Winston.

Rowley, D. (1992) Creating a desirable future for people with significant learning difficulties? in G. Fairbairn and S. Fairbairn (eds) *Integrating Special Children: Some Ethical Issues*. Aldershot: Avebury Ashgate Publishing.

Russell, P. (1990) The Education Reform Act – the implications for special educational needs, in M. Flude and M. Hammer (eds) *The Education Reform Act 1988: Its Origins and Implications*. Lewes: The Falmer Press.

Rynders, J., Johnson, R., Johnson, D. and Schmidt, B. (1980) Producing positive interactions among Down's Syndrome and non-handicapped teenagers through co-operative goal structuring, *American Journal of Mental Deficiency*, 85: 268–73.

Sanberg, L. D. (1982) Attitudes of non-handicapped elementary school students toward school-aged trainable retarded students, *Education and Training of the Mentally Retarded*, 17: 30–4.

Sayer, J. (1985) A whole-school approach to meeting all needs, in J. Sayer and N. Jones (eds) *Teacher Training and Special Educational Needs*. London: Croom Helm.

Sayer, J. (1987) *Secondary School for All?* London: Cassell.

Schratz, M. (1993) From co-operative action to collective self-reflection: a sociodynamic approach to educational research, in M. Schratz (ed.) *Qualitative Voices in Educational Research*. Lewes: The Falmer Press.

Shapiro, A. and Morgolis, H. (1988) Changing negative peer attitudes towards students with learning disabilities, *Journal of Reading, Writing and Learning Disabilities*, 4(2): 133–46.

Sharp, R. and Green, A. (1975) *Education and Social Control*. London: Routledge and Kegan Paul.

Sheare, J. B. (1974) Social acceptance of educable mentally retarded adolescents in integrated programs, *American Journal of Mental Deficiency*, 78(6): 678–82.

Siperstein, G. N., Budoff, M. and Bak, J. J. (1980) Effects of the label 'mentally retarded' and 'retarded' on the social acceptability of mentally retarded children, *American Journal of Mental Deficiency*, 8(4): 596–601.

Siperstein, G. N., Bak, J. J. and O'Keefe, P. (1988) Relationships between children's attitudes towards and their social acceptance of mentally retarded peers, *American Journal of Mental Retardation*, 93(1): 24–7.

Slee, R. (1993) The politics of integration – new sites for old practices? *Disability, Handicap and Society*, 8(4): 351–60.

Speier, M. (1976) The child as conversationalist, in M. Hammersley and P. Wood (eds) *The Process of Schooling*. London: Routledge and Kegan Paul.

Stainback, W. and Stainback, S. (1981) A review of research on interactions between severely handicapped and non-handicapped students, *The Journal of the Association for the Severely Handicapped*, 6: 23–9.

Stainback, W. C., Stainback, S. B. and Dedrick, C. V. (1984) Teachers' attitudes toward integration of severely handicapped students into regular schools, *Teacher-Educator*, 19(3): 21–7.

Stillman, A. (1990) Legislating for choice, in M. Flude and M. Hammer (eds) *The Education Reform Act 1988: Its Origins and Implications*. Lewes: The Falmer Press.

Strain, F. (1984) Social behaviour patterns of non-handicapped and developmentally disabled pairs in mainstream pre-schools, analysis and intervention, *Developmental Disabilities*, 4(1): 15–28.

Stratford, B. (1985) Learning and knowing: the education of Down's Syndrome children, in D. Lane and B. Stratford (eds) *Current Approaches to Down's Syndrome*. London: Holt, Rinehart and Winston.

Strully, J. and Strully, C. (1985) Friendships and our children, *Journal of the Association for Persons with Severe Handicap*, 10(4): 13–16.

Swann, W. (1985) Is the integration of children with special needs happening? An analysis of recent statistics of pupils in special schools, *Oxford Review of Education*, 2(1): 3–18.

Swann, W. (1991) *Segregation Statistics – English LEAs, Variations between LEAs in Levels of Segregation in Special Schools, 1982–1990*. London: Centre for Studies on Integration in Education.

Taylor, R. (1992) *Visual Arts in Education*. Lewes: The Falmer Press.

Taylor, S. and Bogdan, R. (1989) On accepting relationships between people with mental retardation and non-disabled people: towards an understanding of acceptance, *Disability, Handicap and Society*, 4(1): 21–35.

Thomas, D. (1978) *The Social Psychology of Childhood Disability*. London: Methuen.

Thomas, D. (1982) *The Experience of Handicap*. London: Methuen.

Thomas, D. (1985) The determinants of teachers' attitudes to integrating the intellectually handicapped, *British Journal of Educational Psychology*, 55: 251–63.

Thomas, H. (1990) From local financial management to local management of schools, in M. Flude and M. Hammer (eds) *The Education Reform Act 1988: Its Origins and Implications*. Lewes: The Falmer Press.

Thurston, L. L. (1928) Attitudes can be measured, *American Journal of Sociology*, 33: 529–44.

Thurston, T. G. (1959) *An Evaluation of Educating Mentally Handicapped Children in Special Classes and in Regular Classes*. Chapel Hill: School of Education, University of North Carolina.

Tognacci, L. N., Weigel, R. H. and Vernon, D. T. (1974) Specificity of the attitude as a determinant of attitude-behavior congruence, *Journal of Personality and Social Psychology*, 30(6): 724–8.

Tomlinson, S. (1982) *A Sociology of Special Education*. London: Routledge and Kegan Paul.

Tomlinson, S. (ed.) (1994) *Educational Reform and its Consequences*. London: IPPR/Rivers Oram Press.

Towne, R. C. and Joiner, L. M. (1968) Some negative implications of special placement for children with learning disabilities, *Journal of Special Education*, 2: 217–22.

Trieschmann, R. B. (1980) *Spinal Cord Injuries*. Oxford: Pergamon Press.

Uditsky, B. (1993) From integration to inclusion: the Canadian experience, in R. Slee (ed.) *Is There a Desk for Me? The Politics of Integration*. Lewes: The Falmer Press.

Verity, D. (1991) Give and Take, *Zero Three*, 5: 17.

Vlachou, A. (1995a) 'Teachers and peers' attitudes towards the integration of pupils with Down's Syndrome', unpublished Ph.D. thesis. University of Sheffield.

Vlachou, A. (1995b) Images and the construction of identities in a research context, in P. Clough and L. Barton (eds) *Making Difficulties: Research and the Construction of SEN*. London: Paul Chapman Publishing.

Vlachou, A. and Barton, L. (1994) Inclusive education: teachers and the changing culture of schooling, *British Journal of Special Education*, 21(3): 105–7.

Vulliamy, G. and Webb, R. (1993) Special educational needs: from disciplinary to pedagogic research, *Disability, Handicap and Society*, 8(2): 187–202.

Warnock, M. (1978) *Special Educational Needs* [The Warnock Report]. London: HMSO.

Warnock, M. (1991) Equality fifteen years on, *Oxford Review of Education*, 17(2): 145–53.

Webster, F. (1980) *The New Photography: Responsibility in Visual Communication*. Edison, NJ: Whitehurst and Clark.

Weigel, R. H. and Newman, L. S. (1976) Increasing attitude-behavior correspondence by broadening the scope of the behavioral measure, *Journal of Personality and Social Psychology*, 33(6): 793–802.

Wexler, P. (1992) *Becoming Somebody: Toward a Social Psychology of School*. Lewes: The Falmer Press.

Whitty, G. (1990) The new right and the National Curriculum: state control or market forces? in M. Flude and M. Hammer (eds) *The Education Reform Act 1988: Its Origins and Implications*. Lewes: The Falmer Press.

Williamson, B. (1981) Contradictions of control: elementary education in a mining district 1870–1977, in L. Barton and S. Walker (eds) *Schools Teachers and Teaching*. Lewes: The Falmer Press.

Wisman, J. P. (1986) Friendship: bonds and binds in a voluntary relationship, *Journal of Social and Personal Relationships*, 3: 191–211.

Wolcott, H. F. (1977) *Teachers vs Technocrats*. Eugene: University of Oregon, Center for Educational Policy and Management.

Wolfensberger, W. (1972) *The Principle of Normalization in Human Services*. Toronto: National Institute on Mental Retardation.

Wolfensberger, W. (1989) Human services policies: the rhetoric versus the reality, in L. Barton (ed.) *Disability and Dependency*. Lewes: The Falmer Press.

Woods, P. (1977) Teaching for survival, in P. Woods and M. Hammersley (eds) *School Experience: Explorations in the Sociology of Education*. New York: St Martin's Press.

Woods, P. (1981) Strategies, commitment and identity: making and breaking the teacher, in L. Barton and S. Walker (eds) *Schools, Teachers and Teaching*. Lewes: The Falmer Press.

Woods, P. (1983) *Sociology and the School: An Interactionist Viewpoint*. London: Routledge and Kegan Paul.

Woods, P. (1986) *Inside Schools*. London: Routledge and Kegan Paul.

Woods, P. and Pollard, A. (eds) (1988) *Sociology and Teaching: A New Challenge for the Sociology of Education*. London: Croom Helm.

Yuker, H. E. (1988) Perceptions of severely and multiply disabled persons, *Journal of the Multihandicapped Person*, 1(1): 5–16.

Zigler, E. and Hodapp, R. (1986) *Understanding Mental Retardation*. Cambridge: Cambridge University Press.

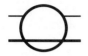

Index